Just Before the Giggle

Just Before the Giggle

A Journey from Suffering to Freedom

Alan W. Weiner

iUniverse, Inc.
New York   Lincoln   Shanghai

Just Before the Giggle
A Journey from Suffering to Freedom

iUniverse books may be ordered through booksellers or by contacting:

iUniverse
2021 Pine Lake Road, Suite 100
Lincoln, NE 68512
www.iuniverse.com
1-800-Authors (1-800-288-4677)

Because of the dynamic nature of the Internet, any Web addresses or links contained in this book may have changed since publication and may no longer be valid.

The information, ideas, and suggestions in this book are not intended as a substitute for professional advice. Before following any suggestions contained in this book, you should consult your personal physician or mental health professional. Neither the author nor the publisher shall be liable or responsible for any loss or damage allegedly arising as a consequence of your use or application of any information or suggestions in this book.

ISBN: 978-0-595-44628-5 (pbk)
ISBN: 978-0-595-69559-1 (cloth)
ISBN: 978-0-595-88953-2 (ebk)

Printed in the United States of America

"I choose to give up suffering."

"… when I am suffering, (I) look to the cause of it in myself, and give up whatever makes me do it, leaving the space wide open to whatever comes in. It isn't easy, but surely is a ladder to heaven.
"Of course, I am giving up luxury—the luxury of feeling sorry for myself.
"… seeing the whole thing clearly.
I burst out laughing."

—Barry Stevens, "Burst Out Laughing" 1984

TESTIMONIALS

"*Just Before the Giggle* is a tremendous accomplishment. It makes hitherto difficult personal growth work easy and accessible to both beginners and advanced meditators. I found the exercises tremendously useful."

—Dr. Raj Secura, Ph.D. Trans-Personal Psychology

"This book is exciting. I found the format of the individual exercises elegant in simplicity and power. The author has a talent for expressing intangible concepts in tangible ways. The book builds on practical experiential reality with precision to provide a window on the unknowable. The result is a demystification of the human condition. Each exercise is doable and I believe will provide an invaluable guide for anyone who is tired of suffering."

—Dr. Linda Bartlett, MD

"Alan's book exposes the deep mystery at the heart of who we are in an easy to understand, safe and palatable way. It should be a source of comfort, hope, and inspiration to many."

—Richard Page, MS, Health Services.

"I love this book. It provides fascinating way to explore our inner consciousness. Alan Weiner packs the essence of a course of hypnotherapy visits into a manual anyone can use to dialogue with their hidden thoughts. The book was a real pleasure to read and I am enjoying the insights I gained while doing the exercises."

—Dr. Barbara Boyer, DO

"Good job, Dad."

—Dr. Ray Weiner, Ph.D. Cognitive Neuroscience

CONTENTS

JB4G

Just Before the Giggle

(JB4G)

Is Dedicated To

My Many Teachers,
Fellow Seekers
and Traveling Companions.

The Surprises We Uncover
On Our Quest
Continue To
Amaze Me.

FOREWORD

I knew Alan Weiner casually for a number of years because we have sons the same age who were attending the same religious studies. I first learned of his hypnotherapy credentials during a weekend family religious retreat, where he was asked to tell our group about hypnotherapy and do a demonstration.

Over the years our families became friends. I found that Alan has led a rich personal life and traveled a very interesting spiritual path.

In 1989 at age 40 I had a catastrophic respiratory illness requiring an extended hospital stay and lengthy rehabilitation. Prior to that time I had been healthy. Although I have made a remarkable recovery I have a number of limitations as a result of the illness and prolonged hospitalization. I also acquired Hepatitis C.

Alan and I had talked briefly about hypnotherapy as vehicle for dealing with pain. In May of 2005 I asked to work with him in preparation for a yearlong treatment for Hepatitis C. Alan had just returned from a hypnotherapy conference. He was excited about his experience there and the many ways hypnotherapy was being used to improve peoples' lives. He was ready to move from a single hypnotherapy visit for a single issue approach (intervention model) to an ongoing exploration process (coaching model). So Alan and I began an amazing discovery process as we explored ways to alleviate chronic pain and fatigue and move toward a state of balance and equanimity.

Our work together was very exciting and we soon recognized what a positive change had come about in my daily life and also in Alan's. Our journey had given Alan incredible insight into a process that could be simply represented and taught to many people in a written format.

Alan has the passion, energy, and genius to simplify life's experiences into clear, tangible, practical exercises. He also has the rare gift of being able to take complex concepts and actually present them in simple understandable visual diagrams. As a fellow scientist I am most amazed and appreciative of this gift and the way Alan uses this to promote learning and understanding. I have struggled most of my life trying to reconcile and find a bridge between my spiritual and scientific natures. To have someone who shares that same struggle is a great comfort in itself. To have that person be able to take the struggle to a level of understanding that I had begun to believe might be impossible, is a true delight.

Through my own journey of personal growth and understanding I had been unable to fully integrate my body, mind and spirit connection. I have had the help of very good teachers who have also been supportive and loving to me in my process. Alan has helped me to finally experience the power, possibilities and comfort that the integration of the body, mind and spirit can bring. In our process we both focused on celebrating joy on a daily basis. We have both been delighted by the wonders and gifts of that celebration.

Linda Bartlett
2007

ACKNOWLEDGMENTS

I would like to thank Dr. Linda Bartlett for her bravery, her willingness to grow and change, and her permission to use her real name in this book.

I would also like to thank my team of reviewers for their diligence and their sometimes brutal honesty. Together we have moved through my rough drafts to this final manuscript. In particular, special thanks go to:

- Dr. Raj Secura, for working through each of the exercises and verifying that they translate into the written word.

- Richard Page, for line-by-line editing for consistency.

- Dr. Elizabeth Weiner, Ph.D. Clinical Psychology, for looking at the manuscript from the point of view of a mental-health professional.

- George Stratton, for repeatedly asking, "How does this section or phrase or word contribute?"

- David Woodard, Rebecca Weiner, and Theodore Bresler, for catching typos and extra words that crept into the manuscript during the rewrite process.

- My wife, Phoebe, for her independence of spirit, her willingness to give me the space to write, and her ability to communicate corrections in loving ways.

And a final thank you to the cover girls, Shayna and Diana Beckerman.

Introduction: What is freedom?

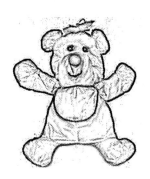

The Journey

This book maps a journey to fully experience aliveness. It supplies the basic tools to carry a person toward balanced, integrated living and freedom from pain.

The Challenge

Would you like to live pain free? Are you willing to suffer less? If a positive, drug-free, alternative exists, are you willing to give up suffering?

Among the tools presented, this book will teach several self-hypnotic healing techniques to help you accomplish your goals. Hypnotic healing approaches pursued by many of my colleagues are based on a belief that a person must return to and fully face moments of suffering to get on with the business of healing. *It is my belief that you have suffered enough!* It is time to give up the drama and experience the divine comedy that is life.

The Learning

Almost twenty years ago Linda, a medical doctor, suffered a serious trauma and, as a result of the injuries and resulting complications, has been in pain ever since. As one would expect, she is well versed in the pharmacological model of pain management, both its positive aspects and its drawbacks. Over the years, multiple therapies had failed to provide sustained relief and had not provided the integration of mind, body, and spirit that she was seeking. In addition, the administered drug levels had been increased to what she considered an unacceptable level.

She approached me and we started a series of hypnotherapy sessions with the goal of mitigating the burden of physical pain. As our sessions progressed, we discovered that our journey was not just about chronic pain, or even about therapeutic healing. It turned out to be an exploration of the human condition.

Each session brought out another aspect of personal growth and our time together became an exploration of what it means to be human, the nature of pain, the nature of forgiveness, the nature of peace, and ultimately, the nature of freedom. What started as a journey away from pain became a journey of discovery; discovery of the quality of life available to all of us in each moment.

As the months passed, our understanding deepened. It became clear that our progress had a definite pattern; a pattern that could be useful for others who strive to be healthier. Eventually, our meetings evolved to become celebrations of life rather than formal therapy. This transcendence became a compelling reason to share our learning.

The Plan

In my clinical hypnotherapy practice, I listen to the disclosure of symptoms. I make no attempt to diagnose an illness based on those symptoms nor do I suggest any medical treatment to cure a disease. Rather, I attempt to convey information about an integrated full-person approach to our situation in life. This approach allows my clients to marshal their inner resources in such a way that discomfort is minimized and an environment for healing is created that can reduce medical or pharmacological intervention.

My clients are able to use the techniques they learn to help themselves be themselves. I hope that the path presented in this book provides you with the tools to alleviate suffering and achieve the full freedom to be yourself.

Each of us has different lessons to learn, and on any path some will intuitively skip a stepping stone or two. In documenting our journey, I have added steps and pulled in information gleaned from addressing many clients' issues as well as dealing with the joys and tragedies in my own life experience. My goal is to include sufficient steps so that everyone may follow this journey.

The Actualization

Chapter One of this book gives a glimpse of the destination (balance) and the way to get there (joy). Why wait to minimize suffering? The next few chapters present modeling information on how the mind works. They cover essentially the information that I would normally present during my first meeting with a client. I explain the nature of human beings as derived from the hypnosis mind-model.

The chapters that follow address balance in different areas of our lives. Each of the sections in these chapters starts by presenting a specific challenge. This is similar to how a hypnosis session starts: "What would you like to work on today?" Then some applicable useful information or insights about the nature of the mind, the body, and their interaction is conveyed. This is the kind of information that would come out of a client-therapist dialogue or trance work. Most sections end with practical exercises that you may perform in order to make the information your own. The intended result is that you develop a new skill or refine a skill you already possess.

Successful therapies come to a conclusion. The last few chapters of this book move on to celebrations of life.

The Practice

We believe that insights we uncovered are universal. I hope that this expression of them will be of benefit to all. Since you are here, reading these words, it is my intent that the concepts and tools be of direct benefit to you. The exercises are directions designed to help you manifest that benefit.

The techniques presented in this book allow my clients to be the kind of people that they are really excited to be. The kind of people they are proud to know and honored to hang out with. I wish this same exuberance of spirit to be available to you.

As humans we constantly maintain an inner dialogue. Among other things, *the specific wording of our dialogue,* unique for each individual, *matters.* Some of the exercises scattered throughout this book are designed to help you get at the heretofore buried assumptions and habit patterns that drive your own internal dialogue. I invite you to do the exercises, clarify your desires, find your key words, and take conscious control of your inner tongue. This will propel you even faster away from suffering and toward freedom.

God speed and welcome home!

About the Therapist

Some of my clients want to know a little about me and my background before we start working together. This section is to address that request. Just skip it if you like.

It seems that I have always thought of myself as a scientist. I have early memories of taking apart a radio, of stars on a clear night, of my chemistry set and my "mad scientist" lab in the basement. My first engineering job was applying computer technology to the efficient and safe generation and transport of electrical power. My career moved into management. I eventually led teams of up to thirty-five people on complex control systems projects.

Trying to understand and motivate my team, I noticed similarities between the way computer programs follow procedures and the way some folk seemed to be locked into specific behavior patterns.

I studied Bandler and Grindler's development of Neural-Linguistic Programming™ (NLP)[1] and applied NLP techniques to supervision. I participated in human awareness seminars and retreats as a staff member and eventually as a speaker. I took formal training and became certified as a Clinical Hypnotherapist by the American Council of Hypnotic Examiners (ACHE). For the past fifteen years I have run a small practice out of my home.

Today I work as a hypnotherapist and as an engineering consultant. My hypnotherapy practice helps me to be of service in the psychological world while my consulting practice helps me to be of service in the physical world. My clients tell me that my ability to accept both worlds at the same

---

1   NLP is covered in more detail later in Chapter 9 when we discuss personal styles and in Chapter 11 when we discuss societal styles.

time helps them to also integrate these seemingly disparate aspects of their own being.

My secret in accepting and balancing the physical world and the psychological world is finding stability in a third world, that of spirit. I've been blessed to find teachers who helped me to uncover, experience, and appreciate some of the unfathomable mysteries that underlie who we are as human beings. Some of my experiences with a particular sage are included in the afterword to this book.

Chapter 1 Figures

Chapter One
Joy

1   THE JOY OF DISCOVERY, THE DISCOVERY OF JOY

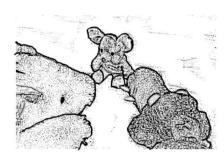

The path that Linda and I took led us to a way of being that has transformed our lives and the lives of those around us who are now experimenting with it. I invite you to join this group of vibrant people. I invite you to experience your life through a filter of joy.

I have noticed that pain and suffering act as indicators that something in my life is not working well for me and needs to be changed. Pain comes to me from my body as a message of physical hurt. Suffering comes to me from my story of myself as a message of emotional hurt. Both messages tell me of situations that I would benefit from changing. In our first sessions, Linda and I gained the insight that pain messages were signals of imbalance somewhere in our lives.

I can consider the pain as a warning message, like a warning light that goes off on a car's dashboard. I can look for the cause of discomfort. If I assume that imbalance is the issue, I can look in all the areas of my life for the current causes of imbalance. As I identify the causes, my creative abilities can come into play to prompt movement, in any area, toward equanimity and peace.

It turns out that humans have a built-in balance-generating mechanism. When a baby is presented with a new situation and it does not know how to react, you can see the puzzlement and worry in its face as it analyzes the situation. If the situation resolves to one of safety and familiarity, the child experiences a moment of relief when all is familiar once again. If the resolution is joyous, the child responds with a giggle of pleasure. If, on the other hand, the situation resolves to one of fear, you have a crying baby on your hands.

Again, notice that you can see the resolution of the baby's inner process to "I like it." as the baby's body language moves from neutral to smile or giggle. And, alternatively, you can see the resolution of its inner process to "I dislike it." as the baby's body language moves from neutral to frown or whimper. The baby can also choose to ignore or not notice the new situation and remain neutral.

The baby's interpretation process in response to a stimulus is pictured in the *Baby's World* box.

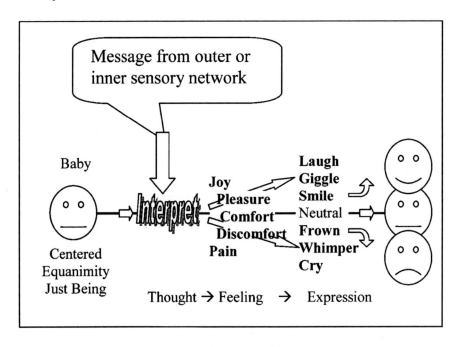

A Baby's World

When people are comfortable they do not think about being comfortable, they are just in that state. When people have been living at a level of discomfort for a long time they are certainly not happy about it, but they have grown accustomed to it. They tend to take that state as normal. Although, as adults they may not always show it, when people are in chronic pain they may live their lives with a constant whimper going on inside them.

If you can add a giggle, by any means possible, you can move the emotional balance point of your experience toward joy and regain a natural sense of equanimity.

It turns out that adding a giggle is not hard. It follows naturally from joy. Just follow the visualization steps in the *Joy Visualization* box on the next page. This visualization is not an intellectual exercise. It is a highly emotional exercise. Let the wonderful, creative child within you, the child who believes that there is magic in the world, have free rein to play in the *Joy Visualization* box. It is a sandbox and the child is safe there.

As adults, we can choose, arbitrarily, to greet any situation we find ourselves in with a giggle. This approach is not meant to be flippant, or to undermine, in any way, the seriousness of our life-situation. Rather, it is designed to allow our creativity to come into play in ways that help us cope with and position ourselves to overcome any adversity.

The *Joy Visualization* box is designed to direct you to a healing place inside you. The joy visualization is about pure joy, not about joy in action. It is not the joy of giving, or the joy of receiving. It is the joy of simply being.

Please remember (or make up) a time when you were joyously deliriously happy, a time when the child in you felt surrounded by love. For simplicity, we will refer to this emotion as "joy." The kind of joy we are referring to is the kind identified in the *A Baby's World* box, the kind that you can sometimes see on a pleased young child's face as you hear the child giggle. This is a starting point for the joy presented in the *Joy Visualization* box.

> Allow yourself to drop through the warm, light blue, transparent sky, feeling the wind support you, celebrating, feeling the *joy*.
>
> Feel the child-like *joy*; wonderment; fulfillment.
>
> Feel the exuberance start in your belly, well up in your chest, and promise to break free.
>
> Experience the *Joy* that comes *just before the giggle*.
>
> Hold yourself just short of the giggle for a time …
> (2 seconds? 10 seconds?) and eventually let the giggle happen.

Joy Visualization

Now that you have a grasp of the emotion, is there a part of your body or your life experience that is currently out of balance? Move the feeling of joy that comes just before the giggle to fill, cover, or surround that place. Let any sore spot in your body be bathed in joy. Let any empty places in your being be stuffed with joy. Enjoy the feelings for as long as you like.

It turns out that this visualization can not only overcome present pain, but can even keep the pain experience from showing up at all. Practice this for a few minutes at a time, and repeat as many times a day as you like. It is an entertainment that seems to have no down side.

My patients and acquaintances have used this visualization while sitting still or in conjunction with Tai-Chi or any low-impact regular exercise. It has been used by some patients in conjunction with devotional exercises.

Linda and I discovered that by utilizing the joy visualization it was possible for Linda to change her way of living. The joy visualization turned out to be a daily practice that could not only transform her experience of pain, but could change her relationship to suffering in a way that automatically moved her toward balance without the need to even experience the pain part.

Steven C. Hayes, a Professor of Psychology at the University of Nevada, Reno, has developed Acceptance and Commitment Therapy (ACT), a therapy that hinges on a distinction between pain and suffering.[2] His thesis is that experiencing painful events is a normal part of the human condition. The effort we expend on avoiding or trying to come to terms with our memories of those experiences drives us into long-term suffering.

I agree with his analysis. However, I have a slightly different way of presenting the mechanism that takes advantage of our way of forming memories to create positive change.

Our memory retention is related to the emotional content of our experience. If we have a strong negative feeling our retention is high but our after-the-fact replay of the event as we try to make sense of it clouds the actual event. The result is that our memory of the event has impact but is not particularly useful. If, on the other hand, we have a strong positive feeling, our memory of the event has both impact and usefulness. This is called learning.

It turns out that the nature of the world is such that over time we tend to accumulate more impact from our negative experiences. We tend to mull over them more and so retain them longer and in more detail. In my experience, many older people seem to have their list of complaints more readily available than their list of joys. Over time the negative memories build up and drag us down into depression. This is shown in the *Regaining Wonder* box. The joy visualization seems to fill our balloon and raise our sprits back toward wonderment.

As time passes our thoughts and memories about the serious events in our lives tend to weigh down our spirit. We

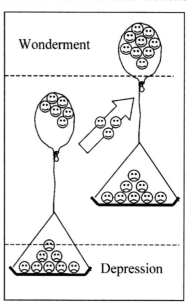

Regaining Wonder

---

2   I particularly like Hayes's book, *Get Out of Your Mind & Into Your Life*. Further information about this book and all other books or web-sources mentioned throughout JB4G may be found in the bibliography.

feel the gravity of our situation. A giggle acts as anti-gravity. It counteracts how seriously we take our situation.

The joy visualization sets the stage for internal healing on all levels. It allows our emotional resources to be energized on behalf of our entire being. It sets the stage for integration of our whole person in an easy and natural way.

Picture the wonder on the face of a baby watching soap bubbles floating in the air. The baby is new to the world, and learning without expectations. The bubbles float and drift, magically suspended. They drift close and the baby sees reflections of the world shimmering in them. One drifts closer and the baby sees his or her own reflection, another baby-face to interact with. Then the bubble pops! Peek-a-boo, and the bubble and the face are no more than a moist breeze. The wonder and mystery turns into a baby's giggle. And we, who are privileged to watch, respond with an inner giggle of our own.

There is a place of healing inside of us, a place of joy beyond words, a place of wonder and mystery that we move through just before the giggle. What would your experience of life be if each moment was lived in that place just before the giggle? Could a giggle be a gateway to enlightenment? I know that the calm that comes to me after a good giggle opens me to compassion for my situation and compassion for others.

Pain is sensation viewed through a filter of fear and aversion. In the space just before the giggle there is no room for fear, there is only the impending giggle. We become free to accept our current experience.

A joyous giggle has the power to transform our experience of living. It can, for the moment, reset our experience of our self back toward the innocence of babyhood. I invite you to explore, to discover, and to giggle.

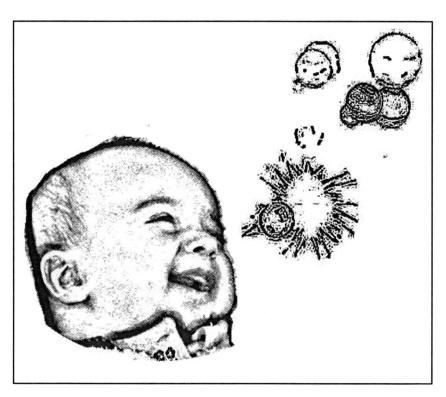

Burst of Joy

Chapter 2 Contents

Chapter 2 Figures

Chapter Two
Understanding

2 Journey Preparation: Knowing Your Mind

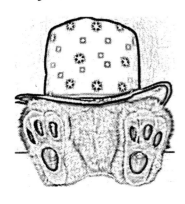 In this chapter, you will discover a useful model of the mind and techniques for learning a new body of knowledge that can ultimately allow you to achieve the freedom that comes from an inner sense of vibrancy. It discusses both the positive and negative sides of memory and personality formation. It introduces concepts to help you through the book and help you through the day. This chapter also provides training in the skills that will be useful in mastering the techniques presented in the following chapters.

This book resulted from a series of hypnotherapy sessions. In my practice, I devote the first session to getting to know my client and providing a little pertinent information about myself. The session continues with establishing the goals for what we want to achieve during the course of the therapy. We also establish the basic tools we will use. We identify our goals and objectives for the therapy. We go into trance together and learn what that feels like. Finally, we learn self-hypnosis to allow us to own and carry forward any insights we gain.

I have organized this book along similar lines. This chapter and the next cover basic concepts and practices that normally come out in our first session. Feel free to read it at your own pace. If I introduce a concept or a practice that you are already familiar with, you may skip it and move on. You can always go back if you need additional practice.

The chapters that follow are organized by topic. Each section represents a particular issue to address. The issue is resolved with the revelation of new knowledge or the reminder of knowledge you already possess. Take your time as you move through these sections. Children grow in the middle of the night as they rest. Take frequent rest breaks to adsorb the new ways of looking at the world that you discover in these pages.

Your self-image is who you think you are. As explained later, it consists of the sum of all the thoughts and feelings that you have experienced and all the decisions that you have made from your first breath until this moment.

Allow the quality of your life to improve steadily over time. You can move as quickly as you like, but *I have noticed that when I change too quickly, I tend to scare my loved ones.* They seem to need more time to adjust to a new me than I need. Be compassionate towards those around you, but do not allow their fears or your own to stop your progress. Most people fear change, even if the change is good. This book is about transformation and change; feel the excitement engendered by the possibility of freedom.

2.1 LEARN LIKE A CHILD

This book is designed to teach you a different way of being in the world, an easy path to pain-managed, or even to pain-free existence.

The easiest way to learn is to learn like a child and one way to do this is to temporarily recapture your innocent-accepting self and absorb useful new concepts just the way that a two year-old absorbs language or a sponge absorbs water.

I contend that the ability to learn quickly, easily, and naturally has a mood associated with it, and if I can recapture the mood, I can recapture the ability. The mood that I find supports easy learning is like being in a safe, accepting, joyous happy place that exists somewhere before a giggle. I successfully ran this experiment during the writing of this book. If I can do it, surely you can do it!

Let's accept that it is possible to learn as quickly as a child. *Remember what it is like to see the world vividly through child-like eyes, to hear sounds of wonder and mystery for the first time, the first taste of apple sauce, the first smell of lilac.*

Your suffering and, in turn, your search for relief has brought you to this moment, to this reading, to this learning. I invite you to play with the concepts, sense what is true for you, and accept who you can become,

When I was first introduced to weight lifting, I was taught, "No pain, no gain." In our present situation let's move from experiencing the pain to embracing the pain and using it for gain. In the next sections we learn and practice a trance state. This state can replicate the innocent accepting space which supports our discovering a new and more fully alive way of being.

2.2   A CHUNK OF PRACTICE

The trance state is useful and natural. We go through it at least two times per day as we transition from outer awareness (awake) to inner awareness (asleep). After we learn something new we need a little time to absorb it. In *Star Wars* after a number of exciting scenes, C3PO said to Luke Skywalker, "Sir, if you'll not be needing me, I'll close down for a while." When we need rest and we feel safe, we naturally fall asleep. In a hypnotic session, a client allows the therapist to become a protective parent, responsible for the physical safety of her body during the session. In this book you are both the client and the therapist so we will take advantage of self-hypnosis to practice and deepen your experiences in useful ways.

A therapist provides several key items during a session:

- A safe environment. We will talk about this more before we actually do any exercises.

- Knowledge of the mind and a game plan that leads toward healing. That is what this book is for.

- A sympathetic ear and a shared experience. You may want to see a counselor for this or make use of your (friends and family) support group.

- Experience and creativity to help the client get at any non-conscious blocks and hindering beliefs. Here I give a plug for hypnotherapists. Your phone book yellow pages will list several in your area under Hypnotherapists or Hypnotists. You might consider seeing one when and if you are so inclined.

When, in your reading, you come across a useful and significant bit of information, you may notice it by a feeling of sleepiness. This could be your mind suggesting a short break to digest the information. This could be an attempt by the part of you that understands learning to drop down into a brain wave frequency where fast learning can occur. Learning is the non-conscious process of creating associations between new data and existing memories. Learning is the process that turns information into knowledge.

Chunking is the mental process of association, integration, simplification, and assimilation that underlies learning.

I experience this moment as a mild sense of confusion. We learn by chunking information and relating or linking the chunks to things we already know. That is why the more you know the more and faster you can learn.

A "chunk" of information is a collection of information that we can hold as one concept. The book currently in your hands is a collection of information that you know now and that you will know later. This meaning and all the interplay of ideas it infers is held as one gestalt or chunk of information that you temporarily label "book" so you can simplify the world enough to make sense of it.

Although you only are holding one book (one concept), at some level you are aware of the specific cover and unique pages, words, and letters all combined into this concept of "book."

Most people can pay attention to seven plus or minus two (7+/-2) chunks of information at a time. The 7+/-2 phenomenon occurs often in nature and science. Search algorithms that optimize width to depth of a decision tree and set up for the best and quickest decision consist of five to nine weighted choices at each level. If you get the warning signal (Feeling sleepy?) that you are holding too many chunks, it is a good time to take a break.

Find a safe place. A safe place is a relatively quiet place free of distractions and interruptions (Is your cell phone off?) where you feel safe and comfortable. A location somewhere in your home is good. A library may work. A bus or train is not so good. Allow yourself around ten minutes of alone-time to read and complete the next few exercises.

Rest your eyes by looking away from the book and take a few slow breaths. Now read the contents of the *Trance Practice 1a* box below, and follow the steps outlined. Your eyes may stay wide open or drop to half open as you read the directions.

Allow your eyes to close at the "..." when you get to the end of the box.

---

1. Look around. Are you in a safe place? Yes.

2. Are you comfortable? Sitting with this book resting in hands, lap, or table? Yes.

3. Take note of the time. You are about to take a five minute break. It that agreeable? Yes.

4. In five minutes the "Chunking" idea will make sense. OK? Yes.

5. Read the next steps and then act.

   a. Slowly breathe in

   b. Slowly breathe out

   c. Allow eyes to close

   d. Notice a sleepy place somewhere in your head

   e. Allow awareness to drop into the sleepy place

   f. Deeper with each breath

   g. Deeper with each breath ...

Trance Practice 1a

Welcome back. Now read the contents of the *Trance Practice 1b* box, and follow the steps outlined.

6. You pop awake with a feeling of pleasant surprise. Yes? *(Any feeling is OK. I happen to like pleasant surprise.)*

7. Notice the time.

8. Less than 5 minutes have passed. Lucky you! Go back to step 5 and repeat breathing for the remaining time.

9. 5 minutes have passed. Good for you! You are starting the process of integrating your conscious and non-conscious minds.

10. More than 5 minutes have passed. Great! You got some extra needed rest. *(I find that depending on what I want to accomplish the eyes closed time runs from 3 minutes to 10 minutes. See what works best for you.)*

11. Feel refreshed? Yes.

12. What does "Chunking" mean?

Trance Practice 1b

If in the above exercise you did not pop awake with a feeling of pleasant surprise or did not eventually feel refreshed, I invite you to run the exercise again. With just a little practice, you can learn to allow the swirl of your thoughts to give way to peace.

2.3 USEFUL TRUTH

You picked up this book as part of a quest to improve your quality of life. Our minds are charged with the protection of our body and to do that we continually learn about the world around us. We continually struggle to distinguish between truth and falsehood.

As adults we have established filters that pretty much sort everything we hear or see as either true or false. There is a middle ground where we take on the attitude of, "I don't know, let's wait and see." The wait-and-see attitude allows us to suspend belief.

The useful flip side of this is that we can use the wait-and-see attitude to suspend disbelief. The ability to suspend disbelief allows us to enjoy a book, movie, or play. The more we suspend disbelief, the more we can drop into the story and feel the emotions portrayed by the characters.

You have probably noticed that the closer new information is related to what you already know is true or what you hope is true, the easier it is to accept.

If new information fits my existing world view I stay well within my comfort zone. The more comfortable I am with new information, the less likely I am to actively question it. This means that it is easy to drop into a world I think I know, each new piece of information layered on the last piece learned.

Many of our basic beliefs are unlikely to be fully thought out. What if something basic to my world view is wrong? Then I may end up buried under a mountain of misinformation. If I look at my basic assumptions about life, it seems that I can either stay complacent and possibly mistaken, or I can question everything and always feel that I am on shaky ground.

Seekers and students of life, such as those who read self-help books, in their quest for improvement attempt to learn what is true for them, how to distinguish truth from fiction and how to test and validate it. This book will be exposing you to some new truths. To help you absorb them, I would like to introduce you to the concept of the Useful Truth.

A Useful Truth is a realization that may or may not be true, but is manifestly useful. Useful Truths allow me to affect my experience of reality. They can provide a handle to hold and transform my relationship to myself and the world. Some Useful Truths are:

- My mind exists to aid my survival in the world!

  Since I know that happy people seem to live longer and healthier lives than sad or depressed people, it may be good for me to use my mind to make myself happy. (This book is full of techniques to do just that!)

- I may not have control over everything that happens to me (Stuff Happens!), but I do have control over how I feel about what happens to me.

Some people accept this as true and others do not. Those that believe this tend to choose positive moods and spend less time in depression than others. If I notice that I have a choice about my mood, I might as well pick a mood that allows me to be effective in the world, or at least allows me to enjoy my ineffectuality.

- Most people are basically good and almost nobody is out to get me!

The world in general is indifferent to my plight and my circle of friends is actively interested in aiding me. Occasionally I run across a sick person or group of people who seem to get their pleasure from causing pain. If I generously assign them the motive of indifference and then avoid them, I get to put energy into addressing my own problems and not waste energy in taking part in a pain drama with them.

- I am alone inside my head!

This gives me privacy and freedom regardless of my circumstances. The me that I am alone with is my past. I can mull on it and curse all that got me to this moment, or I can be thankful for it and use what I have learned to plan for better moments in the future.

- Everything happens for a reason and it serves me!

Most people have trouble believing that this is true. How can I reconcile this Useful Truth with all the stories I know of bad things happening to good people? The point is that it may not be true, but people who act as if it is true find the strength to move on with a positive attitude regardless of what has befallen them. The positive attitude helps a person find the inner creativity to turn their situation around.

- Short learning breaks allow me to sort and integrate new knowledge!

This is most likely true (see chunking in the previous section). It helps me to go easy on myself when I am trying to absorb a new concept. It sets me up to quickly, easily, and naturally expand my knowledge of the world and of myself.

I invite you to run the experiment of accepting a Useful Truth as true for a time and experience how your life may be improved. But first a short break.

---

1. Look around. In a safe place? Yes.

2. Are you comfortable? Yes.

3. Take note of the time. You are about to take a five minute break. Is that agreeable? Yes.

4. In five minutes the "Useful Truth" idea will make even more sense. OK? Yes.

5. Read the next steps and then act.

   a. Slowly breathe in

   b. Slowly breathe out

   c. Allow your eyes to start to close

   d. Notice a sleepy place somewhere in your head

   e. Allow awareness to drop into the sleepy place

   f. Deeper with each breath …

6. You pop awake with a feeling of pleasant surprise.

7. Notice the time.

   a. Less than 5 minutes have passed. Lucky you! Go back to step 5 for the remainder of your break.

   b. 5 minutes have passed. Good for you! You are starting the process of integrating your conscious and unconscious minds.

   c. More than 5 minutes have passed. Great! You got some extra needed rest.

8. Feel refreshed? Yes.

9. Can you tap into that creative part of yourself and make up or recall a "Truth" that is particularly useful to you?

Trance Practice 2

2.4   FINDING THE FICTION

This section starts to address mental pain and anguish. Later sections will address physical pain.

Every story we tell ourselves contains a fiction. We all have a tendency to be at the center of a self drama. From our point of view the world revolves around us. Since the drama is about us, we make it compelling. Like in any good novel, the protagonist has a fatal flaw and a mystery to discover and resolve. Similarly our story contains a fiction that is useful to maintain the drama and suffering.

If my story involves someone else there is even more opportunity to, knowingly or not, add fiction and increase the drama. This drama may be negative or positive. Is this the appropriate time for me to tell you about how uniquely cute, precocious, and adorable my grandchildren are?

If I can identify and give up the unnecessary fiction(s) within my story, there is a possibility for the self-induced suffering to simply evaporate. Now the story may no longer be as interesting or as compelling, but it is also no longer as painful to tell or to live with. Buddhists maintain the Useful Truth, "Suffering is illusion."

I know some people who seem to enjoy their suffering. I can almost picture them rubbing their hands together in glee and they settle down to share a good complaint! Just as a Useful Truth helps us to live more fully, in many cases there might be a Useful Fiction or delusion that helps us inflict suffering on ourselves and on the people around us. I do not think that any of us really do this on purpose. I think that as children we observe behaviors that define ways to be adults in the world. We unconsciously tend to carry these behaviors forward into our adult life, regardless of their actual usefulness in making that live full and meaningful.

I think that if a child grows up in a household where the adults spend their time complaining to each other, that child will spend a good portion of his adult time complaining because that is what he thinks constitutes adult behavior.

It makes sense that in a free or natural state no part of us, including our mind, wants to be in pain. We naturally move away from pain and toward pleasure. I assert, as a Useful Truth, that whenever we are in mental pain there is an underlying not-so-useful fiction. If we can identify the fiction and replace it with a Useful Truth, our world can turn immediately from hell into heaven.

For example:

> Jane is in great mental anguish. She has to declare her aged
> father incompetent and put him into a nursing home. Her
> feelings have her paralyzed into inaction. She is stressed to
> the breaking point when we talk.

The underlying fiction is that he is the daddy and she is the daughter. The Useful Truth is that, from the point of view of care giver, now she is the responsible parent. From that position she can recognize that Dad is no longer able to care for himself or even to be alone for any extended period. This state of affairs frightens him and he acts out based on his fear. He will say and do hurtful things just the way a young un-socialized child might. She is acting out of compassion and doing what is best for him, just as years ago she did what was best for her children when they were too young to judge for themselves.

When she is in touch with her motives and her compassion, the decisions and actions move from impossible to natural. Instead of the image of tough love, where she holds herself as hard-hearted and stiff in her resolve, a new image appears:

> Jane is soft and yielding like a pillow. She can meet each
> of dad's verbal attacks softly and enfold them just the way
> a pillow would. She can do what needs to be done and be
> unaffected by his actions. She can enfold and support him,
> protecting him from the world and himself. She does not
> need to be in stress in any way. Rather, she can be in touch
> with her nurturing nature and grateful for the chance to be
> of service.

A situation that none of us would welcome has been transformed. Such is the power of the Useful Truth.

2.5   HYPNOSIS MODEL OF MIND

It is useful to conceptually split the mind into two parts. Each part has a unique set of tasks and abilities that help it perform those tasks. In this book, we will call the two parts of the mind the conscious mind and the non-conscious mind.

Your conscious mind consists of everything that you are aware of in this moment, while your non-conscious mind contains everything else. Your conscious mind is limited to holding the 7+/-2 chunks of information we discussed earlier, while your non-conscious mind performs massive parallel processing and has no discernable limit.

In the hypnosis model used in this book, the primary purpose of the conscious mind is to keep us alive. It does this by thinking, planning, and making judgments. Its primary job is to interpret sensory experience. In this hypnosis model, the primary purpose of the non-conscious mind is to store instructions and present data to the conscious mind for review.

As an aside, it seems that our non-conscious mind does have a consciousness of sorts. We may become aware of this during dreaming, in a special type of dream called a lucid dream. In a lucid dream we realize that we are in a dream and continue on with it, perhaps enjoying a flying experience, perhaps living a story while we know that we are actually safe in bed. Dreams work by their own set of rules, much different than the rules of reason and logic used by our normal waking consciousness.

It is instructive to ask, "Which part of me is in charge of the decisions I make?" The non-conscious mind filters the thousands of sensory impressions coming into your brain and presents you (your consciousness) with just a few chunks of information for evaluation. How does it determine what to present? At the same time the non-conscious mind also sifts through the millions of possible related memories that are available from your past and presents you with just a few choice memories to aid in your evaluation. How does it determine what memories are relevant?

For example, while you were reading this, there was a definite feeling of pressure from the chair you are sitting in against your bottom. Were you aware of it? You are now. At the same time there is a pressure of this book against your hands. Were you aware of it? You are now.

If you pay very close attention to the feelings in your neck and your ears you may hear/feel your own pulse. Take a moment. Your heart is always beating. The pulse is always there. Can you notice it? What happened to the feeling of pressure from the chair? Ah, it is back now. Remember, our conscious mind can only hold 7+/-2 chunks of information. If we pay attention to one thing we have to stop paying attention to something else.

The non-conscious mind is able to present appropriate survival information from our environment based on learned, context-based, emotional weightings associated with each input. An unexpected noise will interrupt your current reading until you deal with it, assure yourself that no action is required at this time, and assure yourself that it is safe to continue reading. This learned behavior is a result of remembered similar situations.

What we store in each moment is our current sensory data and our interpretation (at that moment) of the data. Since our interpretation is based on past experience, who we think we are is based on all the experiences we have had and the order in which we have had them.

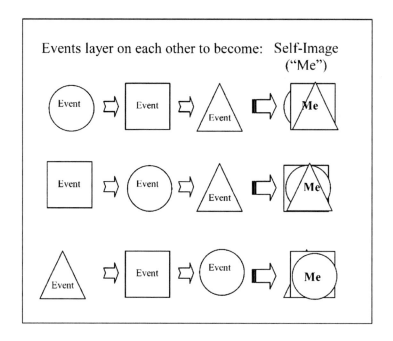

Events Layer to Produce Self-Image

This is a key concept. Take a moment to absorb it. It is depicted in the *Events Layer to Produce Self-Image* box above. The same three events in a different order produce different people. In this analogy, who we are is, essentially, who we think we are, our self image.

We may actually be much more than just our self image. I certainly have resources beyond my current understanding at any time, but what I have specifically available *outside of my self image* remains, for the moment, *outside of my knowledge*. So, effectively, I am my self image.

There are some additional twists that go into making us so interesting:

- The immediacy of events fades over time. New experiences layer on top of old experiences. What I ate yesterday is of more interest to my state of digestion than what I ate last week.

- Each event is weighted by its associated emotional content, so an early emotion-packed event has more effect on our self-image than a newer more neutral event. My aunt would always supply the matzo balls at our family Seder[3]. One year Mom was determined to compete and made her own batch. "How hard could it be?" she said to me as I watched her sweating to make them. I will never forget the dense inedible matzo balls that resulted. They sat at the bottom of the soup tureen. I could not dent one with the side of my fork. My aunt showed up with her matzo balls, which were so light that they seemed to hover in the bowl just over the soup. My uncle suggested that we eat my aunt's matzo balls and save my Mom's to use after the meal as poker chips for a family card game. As I carried Mom's matzo balls back to the kitchen, Dad said to be careful. If I dropped one on my foot, he would have to take me to the hospital. The gathered family howled with laughter and I saw a look of bemused joy on Mom's face as she good-naturedly joined in. I learned, "Do the best you can and enjoy the outcome." Thanks, Mom.

---

3 A Seder is the Jewish Passover meal that celebrates freedom and the exodus from Egypt. It commemorates the biblical story of the night that the angel of death passed over Jewish houses and spared the Jewish first born.

- We interpret events in the light (shape) of earlier events, so we usually fail to see the world as it is. People who did not grow up with my ethnic heritage are unlikely to ever appreciate gefilte fish[4] the way I do. As the taste fills my mouth, I remember the look of pleasure on Dad's face when he tasted it. I remember the family pride in my grandfather, who every year made his gefilte fish from scratch for the Passover meal.

- We interpret ourselves in terms of our actions, so how we may have reacted to events in our past has a great influence on how we react to new events.

- A strongly emotional event can block out earlier events. A little accidental food poisoning kept me away from a particular restaurant chain for years.

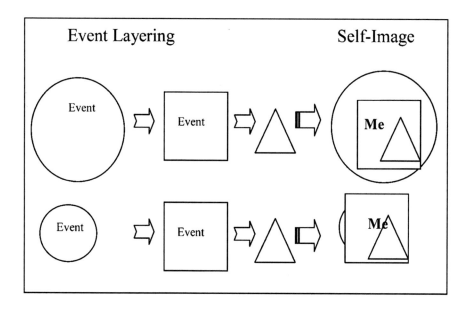

Emotionally Big Events Drive Self-Image

---

4   Gefilte fish is a Jewish ethnic food traditionally made from ground up and boiled whole fish. The fish is mixed with matzo meal and jelled. It is served at Passover with a horseradish topping.

Each event is interpreted in the light of past events and given a weighting based on the emotions associated with those events. Very early events or any new events that are outside of our experience are weighted based on:

- Any physical pain or pleasure being experienced by our body during the event.

- Any physical reactions to the situation by other people around us during the event. This includes facial expression, shouting, laughing, crying, running away, etc.

- Any story people tell us just before, during, or immediately after the event. "This same thing happened to my dead uncle."

We interpret the events around us based on what we know, which is, for the purpose of this model, what we are. The interesting thing about this interpretation mechanism is that it tends to take place *below our awareness*. This means that over time the world around us tends to reinforce the beliefs that we already possess regardless of whether or not the beliefs are justified.

We all have a mixture of "glass is half-empty" people and "glass is half-full" people in our lives. I have had some clients who say things like, "I always respond to adversity with increased determination." and other clients who say things like, "I always respond to adversity with anger or tears of frustration." Although one way seems more useful than the other, both ways are somewhat limiting. I like the more freeing statement, "I tend to respond to adversity with increased creativity!"

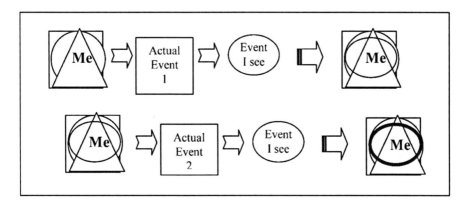

Self-Image Affects Perception

As thinking beings our behaviors result from how we perceive our self interacting with the world. Our observations of our own behavior tend to reinforce the self image that produced that behavior, in many cases, regardless of outcome.

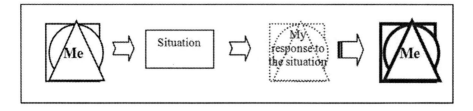

Actions Affect Self-Image

I invite you to consider that although you may think that you have to act a certain way in response to an event, you may actually have many choices, perhaps bounded by your sense of integrity. Given enough time, you are always free to creatively consider all the possible choices in how you deal with a situation.

I have known people who condemn themselves to ineffectual actions with the excuse story, "That is just who I am and I cannot change." You have the freedom to do what you think is right and not be limited by who you think you are, or think you should be. A slight variation of one of the Useful Truths presented earlier is, "I may or may not have any control over what happens to me, but I have total control over how I respond to what happens to me."

Change is always possible. As you change your responses in the direction of life-affirming words and actions, the people in your circle of friends start to see a new you, and, more importantly, each time you react in a new way, you see the possibility for a new you emerging. There is no reason for this process to result in blame, "should-haves," "could-haves," or "would-haves," or for you to take on any onerous penance. Your life gets to become a growth process where each day you become more the person you want to be.

2.6   ONE-TIME LEARNING

Our natural response to strongly emotional events suggests another avenue to one-time learning. Pack the event with a strong emotional charge.

I will never forget my several bone-breaking incidents, and I have learned enough not repeat those disasters. The one-time learning examples that come to mind for most people are usually traumas (negative life-threatening events). However this effect works just as well for positive events. The first time a person holds a new baby and looks into its eyes, their world changes forever, irrevocably and gloriously.

Do you have a favorite memory of a positive event in your life? The memory is of an event that only happened once, but is still vivid and immediate in your mind. I assert that almost all learning and subsequent recall can take place easily and naturally, like experiencing and later recalling a happy event.

Much research has been done that relates multiple factors to learning ability and long-term retention. Much of this research flies in the face of my assertion. I agree that almost all of us will fall short of instantaneous learning and complete retention. However, it is useful to experiment in our own lives. It seems obvious that the more lessons I can learn the first time, the fewer lessons I will have to repeat.

The *Effect of a Traumatic Event* box shows an event traumatizing me and creating a number of new emotional "buttons" that immediately affect how I relate to the world.

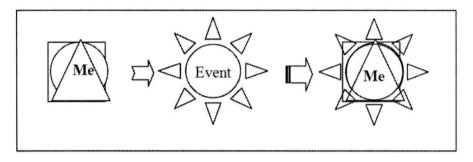

Effect of a Traumatic Event

This is a great survival mechanism and I am glad to have it, but I would like a little more control over who I am and who I am becoming.

Most of us realize that events are subject to distortion, misinterpretation, and misremembering. Emotional cues from others are subject to mis-

Optical Illusion

understanding and conscious or unconscious manipulation by their senders. Verbal stories that are used to place information or an event in context are subject to both manipulation and misunderstanding by their tellers and by their listeners.

The nature of my interaction with the world is such that, I can only see what is in front of me and I never get the whole story. Is this a goblet or two people facing each other? It depends whether I focus on the dark or the light.

2.7 WHAT A FINE MESS WE HAVE GOTTEN INTO

The way the mind works is quite effective for survival. It has successfully gotten you to this moment. The problems with the mechanism are in the area of fine tuning. In the next chapter, I will provide you with tools to take advantage of the mechanism to grant yourself space and the light of self-knowledge.

It takes a relatively accurate on-the-spot interpretation of experience to maintain an adult-level conscious mind. It is generally believed that a child needs to be seven or older to have gleaned enough background knowledge for proper interpretation of day-to-day events. Of course, we may never be prepared for truly traumatic events. At any age, but particularly during our early years, our perceptions are distorted by our *unperceived* inability to grasp the full context of a situation. Remember, as discussed in section 2.4, every story may contain a fiction that helps to give it drama, but also may distort it.

For example, a child stung by several bees, may hear the story, "This same thing happened to my dead uncle." and assume that the stings killed the uncle. This would later result in a fear of bees well in excess of their actual danger. (The uncle may have died of old age years after his bee-sting incident.) This misinterpretation is not useful and does not support survival.

The mind does not like discomfort, so another survival mechanism comes into play that augments our predicament. When a painful event occurs we tend to store it with two instructions to the subconscious:

- Keep me away from anything that looks like this event.

- Block conscious access to the memory of what happened so I do not have to be uncomfortable.

The result is that we move though life avoiding situations without retaining conscious access to the reasons why. We find ourselves in scary situations without knowing why we are scared.

Here is one more example to drive the point home. A child is two years old and playing on the floor. A spider wanders within reach and the child becomes interested and starts to move toward it. At this moment an adult sees the situation.

The adult overreacts and picks the child up quickly enough to inadvertently shake and scare the child. Then the adult stomps on the spider, producing a loud noise which further scares the child and leaves a gooey, hairy spot on the floor.

The event is now a trauma which may be stored by the child with the instructions:

- Hairy = scary
- Forget about it (Hide it from me.)

Years later the child may become an adult that has an unreasonable fear of spiders or may be unaccountably uncomfortable around men with beards. (Yes, it can be that silly!) We end up carrying around misinterpreted experiences and inaccurate information that we do not know about or have access to.

In the next section we consider formal hypnosis and self-hypnosis as a way of gaining access to buried memories that may contain misinformation and may be blocking our experience of living.

Chapter 3 Contents

Chapter 3 Figures

Chapter Three
Training

3 JOURNEY PREPARATION: TRAINING YOUR MIND

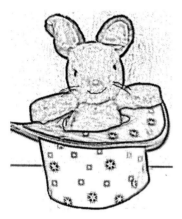

In this chapter, we look at clinical hypnosis and self-hypnosis. We learn about the tools we need to move forward on our journey to achieve balance in our lives. We practice the techniques that will ultimately lead us from suffering to freedom.

I define hypnosis as a state of relaxed, focused awareness where the distinction between awake and asleep, conscious and non-conscious, becomes blurred.

It is a natural state which we all go through at least twice a day when we go to sleep or wake up, but it is not limited to just those times. Some of you reading this may be passing through this state right now. During professional hypnosis sessions another person is involved. In this book we focus on self-hypnosis.

Since you are reading this at your own pace and interpreting the words through your experience, you are in charge. This book is designed to provide you with practical tools to manage pain; it is designed to help you stay consciously in charge of your experience. Through the course of reading and absorbing this book, you will learn self-hypnosis.

Self-hypnosis will allow the conscious you to interact more cleanly and effectively with the non-conscious you. The resulting integration will provide you with pain control and pain reduction, as well as open the door to potential healing and increased aliveness.

3.1   CLINICAL HYPNOSIS

In clinical hypnosis, we have a tool that allows us to go back to the events that formed our self-image. In the case of a traumatic event, we have the chance to bypass the instruction to forget (actually an instruction to not remember) and fully emotionally relive or abreact the event. We have access to the full memory because in the hypnotic state, we are not strictly conscious. The thinking part of us is at rest and does not have to be protected.

When we relive the event there are several significant differences:

- This time we are not alone. We are sharing the experience with the hypnotherapist who is a concerned listener.

- This time we have the knowledge that however scary the event was to the child, we did survive it. We are here now.

- This time we have at our disposal the full set of experiences that continued to form us from the event until this moment. We can use this additional information about the world to re-interpret the event, to gain perspective.

The result is that we now have the knowledge to more accurately access the event we experienced in more positive, life-affirming ways. (Useful-Truth: Everything that has ever happened to me is useful because it has prepared me for and gotten me to this moment.) *The important thing to notice here is that although we cannot change the actual events that transpired; we can modify our emotional relationship to what transpired.* We are doing this in the light of additional information.

For example:

> This afternoon I was attempting to turn left from a side street onto a busy main road. Traffic was clear in both directions, but my turn was blocked by a minivan standing motionless in the middle of the main street left turn lane. The left turn signal was blinking and the driver was talking away on her cell phone. Since she had the right of way, I waited, and waited, and waited.

Finally, convinced that she was brain dead, I took a chance and completed my left turn. As I drove away, I considered capping our interaction with a well-earned hand gesture. I looked back at her in my rear view mirror. The minivan had its warning flashers on, rather than just its left turn signals. The woman was stranded in a dead vehicle and probably calling for help. My limited viewpoint had caused me to draw a totally wrong set of conclusions.

A little more information results in a substantially different perspective. Our goal in modifying our self-image is not to delete any memories, but to augment them with positive associations. We will be a happier people for it.

Who we are today is a layering of who we were at each moment of our past. We have available all the mental states we have ever experienced.[5] A useful tool for successful hypnosis sessions is to become again as a little child.

My theory as to why clinical hypnosis works to facilitate change is related to the way children experience the world. A child is trying to understand a big scary world and has to be protected from the dangers of that world. The child knows this and relies on the adults around it to provide this protection. The child falls asleep trusting that the adults will protect it through the night. The key to the relationship is trust.

The successful hypnotherapist establishes a rapport with the client. This rapport, in turn, allows for trust. The hypnotherapist can now, for a time, take on the burden of vigilance and protect the client from the world. When the client realizes that he is in a safe place, he can drop his own vigilance and "fall asleep." The gateway to the trance state opens.

3.2 GOAL SETTING

Since this is a self-help book, when you started reading you may have had a goal in mind. Let's take a moment to clarify that goal. Now that you

---

5 Remember "Events Layer to Produce Self-Image" on page 27.

have been exposed to the basic operation of the mind, allow me to be your coach.

We need to set a goal so that we have a way of noting our progress toward it. If we write down the goal, we can periodically check back and see where we are in relation to it.

One of several things may happen:

- We notice that we are moving toward achievement of the goal. Great, keep up the good work.

- We notice that we have achieved our goal. Fantastic, celebrate and then it is time for a new goal.

- We notice that our life situation has changed and the goal is no longer important to us. Fine, time for a new goal.

- We notice that the goal is still important, and yet we seem to have made no progress toward it. In fact, we may have made progress in a different direction. We have made a lot of progress in getting nowhere. This may be because:

  o We may have picked a goal that we are actually not all that interested in achieving. Time to clarify and set another goal. (There is a section on how to do this later.)

  o We may be sabotaging our own efforts because we have a hidden agenda, an underlying desire that is in conflict with what we think we want. See (a) above.

  o We may be attempting to proceed in a way that we do not yet have the skills or tools to accomplish. Try a different approach to the goal or try to develop the relevant tools. Insights, tools, and approaches to help you proceed are scattered throughout this book.

For now it is important just to take a stab at what you would like to get out of this book. This is a first pass effort, so do not worry if you do not state what you want to your satisfaction. You can always change your goal. I will not criticize you. It is not about getting it right, it is just about getting it written down.

3.3 SO, WHERE ARE YOU?

Part of setting a goal is to assess where you are now. I use a check list to help my clients prepare for their first session. Take your time to consider the questions. Mark your answers here or on a separate sheet of paper. It may be useful to hold onto the paper as you move through this book.

What motivated you to pick up and purchase this book?

_____

_____

What is your purpose in reading this book at this time?

_____

_____

Indicate any conditions or health afflictions that you may wish to change:

_____

_____

_____

Compelling reason(s) to change:

__ Alcohol Abuse
__ Allergies
__ Blood Pressure too High
__ Blood Pressure too Low
__ Chronic Fears
__ Chronic Good Humor
__ Depression
__ Diabetes
__ Eating Disorder
__ Financial Distress
__ Headaches
__ Hypoglycemia
__ Insomnia
__ Lack of Confidence
__ Learning Disabilities
__ Low Self-Esteem

__ Over Sleeping
__ Pain in Joints
__ Pain in Stomach
__ Pain in Muscles
__ Pain in Teeth
__ Pain in Joints
__ Pain in Sinuses
__ Pain in Back
__ Pain in Butt
__ Pain in (None of My Business)
__ Phobias
__ Relationship Problems
__ Smoking
__ Stress
__ Interested in Being the Best Me I Can Be

Did I miss any that you want to add? Please consider any other situations or conditions you feel are pertinent:

_____

_____

_____

Are you currently under the care of any physicians? If so, for what purpose? (It is always good to review the paid professional members of your team.)

_____

_____

_____

_____

Are you currently in a committed relationship? (It is always good to review and acknowledge the volunteer members of your team.)

_____

_____

If you were to select something to change, what would it be? Write it as a wish here. If you cannot limit yourself to one item (I usually can't), then make a list of items and rank them:

_____

_____

_____

_____

_____

_____

If you do not have anything in your present life that you want to work to change, think about this for twenty-four hours. If you still do not have anything you want to change, please put this book back on the shelf. Someone else may find it useful.

In the next section, you will find some tools to help you grant your wish(es) by bringing a level of self-integration and additional wisdom to your situation.

3.4   MEDITATION

Meditation is a self-induced trance state that has been practiced by folk through the ages to bring peace, calm, and tranquility into their lives. It is similar to a hypnotic trance except no one else is present (clearly a useful prerequisite for exercises that you do when by yourself reading a book).

One fact that you should know about the trance state is that it is close enough to the sleep state that one may, from time to time, drift into sleep. So the down side of a meditation session is some additional rest.

If you are new to meditation the following exercise is a good introduction. If you are an accomplished meditator the following exercise is a good refresher.

I invite you to find a comfortable chair in a secure area.

- Do you trust that you will not be disturbed?
- Do you trust yourself to be alone for twenty minutes?

I invite you to take a moment and access your state of mind-body.

Accessing … Still accessing … Still … Ready to be still …

Please take note of the mental/emotional/physical state you find yourself in.

Good. We will do the exercise itself in a few minutes. First I would like to give you some additional information.

We define ourselves through our thoughts. Just as these words are visible, written in black ink against the white paper, thoughts are audible to our inner ear against the silence of our mind, and pictures are visible to our inner eye against the blackness of our closed eyelids. I invite you to just look for a moment at the blank white between lines or in the book margin. Notice the calming effect of this wordless view. In the same way, just experience for a moment the blank between the pictures in your mind, the silence between the thoughts in your head. It is interesting to ask, are you better defined by your thoughts or by the silence? Some folk say that God speaks in the silence between thoughts, manifests to the quiet mind.

The exercise we are about to do takes about twenty minutes. If you like you can set a timer or just place a clock where you can see it.

Your job for the next twenty minutes is just to breathe. You are quite good at this and have never missed a breath since the moment of your birth. So the idea is to notice that you are breathing in and eventually notice that you are breathing out. If a thought comes up, let it go for now. The twenty minute time frame is a "works for most folk" best suggestion. Beginners generally find that just five or ten minutes works best and long time meditators find that thirty minutes or more is better. I started directly with twenty minutes thirty years ago and I am still happy with that duration.

Most folk beginning meditation find that a lot of the twenty minutes is spent thinking about trying not to think. Some disciplines give practitioners a special word or mantra to repeat. This means that for many of us most of the twenty minutes is spent thinking about how we are not thinking the mantra. But, in any case, somewhere during this time the mind will be silent, if even for just a moment.

The more one practices the more one gets good at finding the inner silence. For me, after thirty years of practice, sometimes the twenty minutes are an eye-blink. Sometimes the first thought is, "Welcome back." I do not know where I went, but I am a kinder, gentler, more open and caring, receptive person for having taken the journey. I tend to like the person who came back even more than I liked the person who left. It will probably take you much less time to reach this state than it has taken me.

Many folk get taken up by the pressures of life and forget for a time about the silence. I recently had the blessing of looking into the eyes of a two-day old baby; the silence is both basic and profound.

When I find that my thoughts are jumbled and I do not seem to know what next to do, I stop for a few minutes, breathe, and look at the blank page that is me. Clarity eventually comes, and I know what to do next.

Read over the steps and try the exercise in the *Breath Meditation* box now … After you have completed the exercise, continue reading at the next paragraph.

Hang out here in this space for a while. Notice if you move out of your peaceful quiet state. What moved you? What thought came up? Were you attached to it? Notice that you are free to entertain your new thought or you may be free to go back to the sense of peace.

Although the *Breath Meditation* process generally takes from ten to thirty minutes, there is a short cut available. A few sections from now, we will practice a technique that will allow us to find inner peace almost anywhere and almost within a heart beat.

---

1. Verify that you will not be disturbed for a while.

2. Get comfortable, sit in a relaxed position. Allow your eyes to close. Shiver once to settle your body.

3. Notice the breath … in … out …

4. Notice a thought. Is it about time?

   • No, go to step 3.

   • Yes, go to step 5.

5. Open your eyes and check the time. Has twenty minutes or more passed?

   • No, close your eyes and go to step 3.

   • Yes, go to step 6.

6. Welcome back. How do you feel? Please continue reading or make notes about your experience.

Breath Meditation

3.5   MODEL OF THE MIND AS RELATES TO PAIN

Pain transmitted from the nerves in the body is received as messages within the brain and interpreted against the inner map of the body (our body image) by the unconscious mind. The unconscious mind then makes a decision, based on previously programmed and inherited parameters, whether or not to pass the information along to the conscious mind. Then we wake up to an "Ouch!" that we get to deal with.

Childbirth appears extremely painful, judging from the reports of many women I know and from my own experience of being present for the births of my children. This particular pain is pain-with-a-purpose! The pain is a by-product of bringing a new human onto the planet. With the purpose in mind, and knowing that her body is designed to succeed at the task at hand, a woman proceeds through the birthing process.

I invite you to notice that the current chronic pain that you may be experiencing may have a purpose. This includes psychological pain. If we can assign it a higher life-affirming purpose, we can address that purpose. Once we have ascertained a purpose associated with some pain, we may be in a position to ask, "How much pain is necessary to achieve the stated purpose?"

Next we will cover several techniques to deal with pain. As the book proceeds things will get even more interesting and, surprisingly, even more simple. There are several conscious pain control techniques, but they work best with the involvement of the non-conscious mind.

3.6   ANCHORS AND SELF-HYPNOSIS

Self-hypnosis allows a person to go into a self-induced trance and retrieve buried treasure (knowledge[6]) from his past. The knowledge gained can give him both the wisdom to accept his present condition and the creativity to find new ways of dealing with it. It is similar to the trance state a clinical hypnotherapist might produce, except no one else is present.

---

6   "…know the truth and the truth will set you free." is a Useful Truth for hypnosis users. It comes from John 8:32.

I remind you that the trance state is close enough to the sleep state that one may, from time to time, drift into sleep. So, as with meditation, the downside of a self-hypnosis session is some additional rest.

It is possible to drop quickly into the receptive, relaxed, introspective state we have been referring to as a hypnotic trance. The mind forms a full image of any event, including sight, sound, smell, external and internal feelings, then tags it for cross reference.[7] We can take advantage of this to bring back a particularly useful state or one similar to it. An example is the meditative state achieved practicing the *Breath Meditation* a few sections ago on page 45.

The following exercise will demonstrate self-hypnosis for relaxation, rejuvenation, and deep rest, as well as mind self-reprogramming. With conscious intent we will lower a finger to drop into trance and eventually raise a fist to return to normal waking awareness, fully alert and rested.

First let's establish a signal or anchor for the wake-up state:

> Sit up straight, head erect, take a breath and let it out. Shiver once to wiggle into your chair. Let yourself feel excited and alive. Raise your right fist into the air—Yeah! Wide awake; Yoo-hoo, Wheee, life is hoot! Root for the home team: the feeling of standing and shouting! **Right fist into the air with intention**; this is your wakeup signal.

Now let's establish the self-hypnotic or trance state: the suggestive state we are looking for is just between waking and sleeping. After you achieve this state, you may use your wake up signal to return to full normal awareness.

Trance State:

> Sit comfortably; shiver once to wiggle into your chair. Let yourself relax. Your back is straight. Your hands rest palms down on top of your legs near your knees. Remember that moment between waking and sleeping—just as you are about to drift away, notice the sleepy place somewhere

---

7   Memory works by like-object association. Any aspect of a memory can cue a re-experiencing of the full memory.

in your head. Let yourself drift. Your jaw relaxes and your head drops easily forward toward your chest. You notice the state ... your eyes naturally close. When you are ready, you raise your fist to return to your normal waking state.

With that trance state in mind, we will establish a signal or anchor to relate to it:

Using the hand you just raised as a fist, touch its forefinger (index finger) to your nose with its three other fingers folded against the palm. The thumb rests against the folded fingers. Holding your hand folded this way rest it on top of your leg near your knee. Your forefinger will be pointed away from you and the other three fingers and thumb of your hand will be resting on top of your leg. Raise your forefinger up until it reaches its natural limit and you feel the tension in the back of your hand. Now, **slowly drop your finger until it rests lightly against your leg.** This is your trance signal. I repeat, your raised forefinger lowered slowly with intention is your signal to prepare for your trance state. Your forefinger resting against your leg is your signal to be in your trance state. If you are not reading directions, as you lower your finger you may lower your eyelids.

Sometimes it takes a breath or two to slow down and prepare for the trance state. You can do this by sitting comfortably; shivering once to wiggle into your chair. And letting yourself relax. Your back is straight. Your hands rest palm down on top of your legs. One hand is closed except for the forefinger, which is raised and pointed forward. You feel the tension in the back of your hand as you hold the finger erect.

Marshal your intention to achieve your trance state. Take a breath in and let it out. As you slowly relax and lower your finger toward your leg you move deeper and deeper into your trance state. As your finger touches your leg you recall the sleepy place somewhere in your head and drop deeply into trance. After a few moments, use your fist-in-the-air signal to come back.

Try this now ... How do you feel?

Now let's practice one more time. This time after your finger touches your leg and you notice your state, raise your finger again and, with intention, lower it down to touch your leg again and notice how your intention drives you still deeper.

3.7   USING SELF-HYPNOSIS

People have a misunderstanding about hypnosis. Because the trance state is close to the sleep state, they think that they have to close their eyes. I recommend dropping your eyelids as you drop your finger. Your lids are closed as your finger touches your leg. Now there is no longer a reason to keep your eyes closed. You can open them and stay deeply in trance, just as a sleep walker moves around with open eyes while remaining asleep. You can open your eyes as needed to read the directions for an exercise while staying deeply in trance and close them as needed if the directions require you to picture something in your mind's eye.

This is all very easy and natural, although it may take a little practice to realize that you are doing it. It turns out that the conscious mind does not really know when the non-conscious mind is in charge and following directions during trance. So from the inside, we cannot always tell that we are in trance. There are subtle differences which we can feel and learn to recognize over time.

Finger-drop exercises end with the fist-in-the-air signal. I suggest that if your eyes are open toward the end of the exercise, close them so that you can open them as you raise your fist into the air.

Among other things, you can use self-hypnosis to:

- **Answer questions:** Write a question down. Drop into trance with the intention of knowing the answer. Come back when you are ready. Later in the day (give yourself at least twenty minutes) look at the question again and see if you have a sense of the answer.

- **Fall asleep at bedtime:** Just turn thinking off, if your mind is still running and keeping you awake.

- **Find peace for rest at bedtime:** Is it possible to use the *Joy Visualization* (page 10) in conjunction with the self-hypnotic finger-drop. Your intention will be to allow the joy to fill any aches and pains that you are experiencing and allow you the peace to naturally drop into deep sleep. Run the experiment. It works for me. It should work for you, if not now, before the end of this book.

- **Augment practices suggested during the rest of this book:** The conscious mind can participate by allowing space for the non-conscious mind to do its job. Times to drop into trance will be suggested. Feel free to use this tool creatively.

3.8   THE VOICES IN THIS BOOK

For the rest of this book, each chapter will deal with a group of related issues that came up for my client, Linda, and may come up for you as stepping stones (or stumbling blocks) on your path toward freedom. Every chapter is divided into sections related to each issue.

Each section represents one hypnosis session with Linda and me. After a brief introduction, an issue is conversationally described under the "Presenting Issue" heading. Linda and I listen to our inner voices to gain wisdom and uncover a Useful Truth that will aid us in dealing with the issue. What we discover is considered and expanded on under the "Dance of Ideas" heading. Finally, you, the reader, get a chance to find your own realization of the Useful Truth that we have uncovered. Exercises designed to help you are suggested under the "Practice" heading.

There are three voices heard in our sessions:

- This normal font is used when I am speaking to you, the reader.

- *An italics font is used when I am speaking to Linda (and you) in a session, and*

- "Indented text in quotation marks" is used to represent Linda's words.

The issues we deal with address a person's relationship with chronic or immediate physical and emotional suffering. In some cases the relationship is direct and obvious while in other cases it may be obscure. The issues all apply to the human condition, but your issues may surface in a different order than presented here. Grab onto what rings true for you and be entertained by the rest. It is my hope that the explorations prompted by this book provide you both immediate and long lasting relief from suffering.

Chapter 4 Contents

Chapter 4 Figures

Chapter Four
Inner Selves

4 BALANCING YOUR INNER SELVES

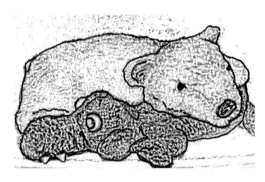

In this chapter we use our pain as a motivator to dive down deep within ourselves. We use it to motivate ourselves to learn more about the events that have gone into our creation. We in no way deny our suffering, rather we take advantage of it as a goad to help us learn more about how we manifest in this world.

4.1 FINDING BALANCE

This session identifies our need for balance in our lives. Suffering of any kind seems to come in cycles. If we identify the suffering as the result of being off balance in some way, perhaps we can interrupt the process.

I invite you to consider the Useful Truth, "If I am not in a state of equanimity, something is out of place in my inner landscape. I am in some way out-of-balance."

I can look within to see what actions, mental or physical, I need to take in order to regain my composure, find my center, and regain stability.

Remember, the Useful Truth may or may not be true. We assume that balance is the issue because getting back into physical balance is something we can do naturally. By extension, finding balance in any other area of our life is something we can own and accomplish.

Presenting Issue:

Good afternoon, Linda. What brings you here today?

> "I am experiencing low energy and nagging chronic pain; it feels like a 'body migraine', the pain comes in waves."

The Dance of Ideas:

I invite you to consider that pain can be used as a driver for communication with the child within you. This child is the part of your non-conscious mind that is linked to and recaptures the creativity and joy of childhood. It is a good ally to have on your journey to freedom.
Please take a breath, bring your finger to your knee, and drop into trance. If your pain could talk, what is it trying to say?

> "Pain can be a reminder to me to keep balance in my life. I see now that it is possible to recognize that I am out of balance before I am so stressed that I trigger a pain episode."

Pain comes in different flavors:

- The pain of a "boo-boo" (small physical trauma) starts fast and drops into background feeling almost as soon as the cause of discomfort is removed. Small burns, needle pricks, scraped knees and elbows; a bandage, perhaps a kiss, and we move on.

- Headaches, backaches, or body aches (from over exercise) may be more bothersome. They tend to last from minutes to hours or even to a day or more.

- The pain of a more serious physical trauma starts soon after an injury as the immediate shock wears off. The discomfort may get worse over time and peak after a few minutes or a few days and then drop off. When I broke my collarbone a few years ago, it seemed that the pain peaked after a few hours and lasted at a surprisingly high level for around a year.

- Some pain is chronic and/or intermittent. The pain of arthritis can seem to be a constant companion, or can come and go like an unwelcome visitor.

Chronic pain as a result of a sustained serious injury or physical situation is usually always with us, but the intensity of our pain varies from mild to excruciating as a function of many factors, such as too much or too little exercise or rest, environmental changes, etc. Fortunately, many of these are at least in part under our own control.

In this section, I present one approach to short-circuiting the usual (pain cycle) pattern where we notice that a chronic pain starts ramping up, and we sadly look forward to a time of misery in our future. The key idea is that chronic pain, which comes in waves, has a slower, more powerful aspect that is like the tide. If we can recognize when the tide is coming in, perhaps we can get to higher ground. The idea is to increase our pain threshold before the pain overwhelms us and we are forced to spend a miserable time-out alone with our suffering or drugged to get through the worst of the pain cycle. It is possible to use a self-hypnosis session to create a pain-recognition early-warning signal. We can then use this recognition signal to take action before our pain threshold is reached and we are immobilized or pushed into increasing our medication to dull the pain.

Consider the following Useful Truths:

- The cycle of pain (either frequency or intensity or both) increases when we are out of balance in some way.
  - We may need more rest than we are getting.
  - We may need more exercise than we are getting.
  - We may need more love or attention than we are getting.
  - We may need less attention than we are getting (i.e., more "space").
  - We may need to give more love or attention than we are giving.
- There is some internal part of us that monitors our stress level and starts the pain ramping up when we get too far out of balance. We can talk to this part of ourselves and negotiate a new signal to let us know that we are approaching the "pain" part cycle. This signal will remind us to take remedial action. We can consciously regain balance before we are forced to do so by the escalating pain messages.

- If we agree to respond to the new signal, and we keep our promise to ourselves, the pain cycle can be bypassed! This means that, for Linda, a two-hour nap taken immediately in response to an early warning signal for rest eliminated a pain episode that would previously have kept her in bed for two days.

Now let's search for your signal. It may be a color you see around you, a vision of some remembered sight, a sound you hear, or an inner voice saying something like, "Watch out" or "Balance." It may be a feeling somewhere in your body, like the pressure of a hand on your shoulder. It may be a special taste, like cloves, or a smell like a hint of sulfur or of jasmine. It may be a combination of things. In any event, it will be unique to you.

Linda found that, for her, the warning signal of impending pain was seeing in her mind's eye, the image of a vivid purple quilt. She found that each time she "saw" the purple quilt it was time to stop and take steps to put herself back in balance. Often for Linda, this meant taking a nap. For you it could mean something else—for example, taking a break from a stressful activity, exercising, or meditating.

The practice paragraphs below provide a short exercise to help you find your early warning signal. For many people, something surprising and unexpected comes up, others at first find nothing in particular. If you do not receive a compelling signal, just make one up. It will do for now. Signals sometimes morph over time.

Practice:

Your intention is to find your early warning signal. I wonder what it could be. Wonder playfully about it for a moment. Some people are most naturally oriented towards the visual (seeing something in our mind), others toward the auditory (hearing something in our mind), and still others to the kinesthetic (the feeling of touching something or of a sensation in our own body). Which are you? Linda saw a purple quilt before her when pain was approaching. My own warning is a voice in my head saying "BALANCE" while I get a feeling in my lower back as if I were trying to walk on a tightrope.

I invite you to:

1. Take a moment to acknowledge the part of yourself that is willing to take responsibility for the pain you are experiencing at this moment and, perhaps, at other times in your life. This part has produced the pain signals to alert you when you have gotten out of balance.

2. Ask this part of you to provide a different signal which you will heed just as you might heed the pain signal.

3. Quiet your mind to receive the signal.

4. Marshal your intention to achieve the trance state; take a breath in and let it out. As you slowly relax and lower your finger toward your leg you move deeper and deeper into the trance state. As your finger touches your leg you recall the sleepy place somewhere in your head and drop deeply into trance. Your head drops forward and your chin rests for a time on your chest.

After a few moments the signal may come to you, use your fist-in-the-air signal to come back. Welcome back. How do you feel?

What is your signal? Write it down.

If you have not come up with a special signal, make one up for now. It can be as playful or serious as you like. You will not be stuck with a particular signal. You can always change it later.

Accept the "pay-attention/wakeup/beware" signal that comes to you and think about how it has meaning in your life, how it is related to balance. Now that you have a warning signal, remember to honor it. A red light does not provide safety if we do not stop.

Sometime, when I have a client who may not have yet identified their early warning signal, I suggest that they temporarily associate Linda's color *purple* with the early pain signal. When we notice that the world around us takes on this *purple* hue (or your identified out-of-balance warning signal), we immediately stop whatever we are doing to heed this early warning. Remember, you are free to translate my signal to your unique inner sound or voice saying a particular word, like "Careful," or "Cuidado," or a unique body sensation, or some combination of thoughts and feelings.

What we are doing with balance is opening a two-way channel of communication between the conscious and non-conscious you. When your wakeup signal appears to you during daily life, stop for a moment and ask yourself, "What do I need to do to achieve balance at this time?" Notice the next thought that comes up and either act on it immediately or schedule a time in the near future to act on it in some way. Then remember to keep your promise to yourself.

To summarize our early warning system practice:

Allow your identified out-of-balance signal to pop into your awareness instead of (in advance of) any pain signals; this message is for you to:

1. Pay attention,
2. Determine what you need to do right now to achieve/maintain balance in your life, and
3. Act on your determination.

Wave to the out-of-balance signal by way of acknowledgment of the message received. Thank the part within you that is providing this warning. If the warning is not heeded, allow your unique signal to become more intense and compelling as necessary to get your attention.

Realize that just accepting the commitment to experiment with this new process is tantamount to change!

If the action toward balance is not possible at the moment when you get the early warning signal, make a specific time and place commitment to take the appropriate action, and keep the commitment. The message that is available here is that the child within learns to weather and survive while the adult within learns to find and maintain balance.

By the way, a person can have more than one signal, and the signals can layer on each other. If I do not acknowledge the first message, "BALANCE" from my non-conscious self, a little later the world around me starts taking on a purple hue, when I see this, I then finally notice the sensation in my lower back and figure out what I need to do to regain equanimity. I thank my non-conscious self for all the signals it sent, both those that I paid attention to and those that I missed.

4.2   LEARNING TO PLAY

I define playing as, "Experiencing the moment and enjoying the experience."

Presenting Issue:

Good afternoon, Linda. What brings you here today?

> "The child within me is afraid to play without knowing the rules."

The Dance of Ideas:

Please drop into trance now. What helpful advice can you give your inner child?

> "Child Linda, you do not have to worry. You can trust me, the inner adult Linda, to watch for appropriateness in the world before we start visibly playing. You are allowed the freedom to play and enjoy the world all the time."

I invite you to consider that since the inner you is totally private, you are free not only to enjoy your world, you are free to laugh at it. No one will ever know how hard you are laughing at the circumstances that make up your life. It hurts no one if you freely enjoy every situation you find yourself in. Consider that if you are your only witness, you may as well laugh your butt off.

The internal laughing approach to all of life has a lot of implications. How upset will I be the next time someone cuts me off while driving? Just how important is the position I am holding in an argument with a loved one? The possibility of always laughing leads to the question, "How can I make it through life as a responsible adult if I do not take things seriously?" My answer is to take everything seriously except myself. My inner reactions are always based (at least in part) on misinterpretation and at best only partial information.[8] My unique viewpoint makes the world both interesting and funny.

This section, and most of this book, suggests helpful things that a person can do when they are alone. Many people, as social animals, question the value of alone time. I suggest that alone time is wonderful and a necessary part of a balanced life. Alone time can allow a person a space of peace in which to recharge and shore up their inner stability.

Practice:

Consider this: when you are alone you are hanging out with someone who is or can become your favorite person, a person who shares your opinion about everything, a person who hears your every thought. A person who appreciates what you have been through and, if not now, most likely by the end of this book, really likes you and is proud to know you and be part of your support team.

I invite you to consider that the concept of full-frontal humor as a consistent approach to life is a gift beyond price. Drop into trance (finger-drop with intention, remember) for a few minutes to fully absorb and appreciate it. It is OK to giggle.

Remember, you marshal your intention to achieve the trance state; take a breath in and let it out. As you slowly relax and lower your finger toward your leg, you move deeper and deeper into the trance state. As your finger touches your leg, you recall the sleepy place somewhere in your head and drop deeply into trance. Your head drops forward and your chin rests for a time on your chest.

After a few moments, use your fist-in-the-air signal to come back. Welcome back. How do you feel?

Here are a few more questions to ponder as you consider balancing your life experience by increasing your internal level of playfulness:

- How will your health be different if you take the actions necessary to create and maintain good health seriously, while, at the same time, you do not take the results seriously? Your actions are under your control, while results are subject to the interaction of you and

---

8   If you have trouble accepting this, go back and review section 2.5.

the universe outside you. What a boring place this world would be if all plans went as anticipated.

- Sometimes it seems that the results we achieve are hardly related to the effort we have expended. A socialized adult, like the person reading this book, has been trained to believe in cause and effect. This is most often a useful approach to life. What does the little child inside that person believe in? Are results caused by divine providence, or mystery, or magic?

- Is it possible to expend effort and behave as if cause and effect are always related, while, at the same time, accepting all outcomes as a gift?

4.3   PLAYING AWAY HEADACHES

The following headache cure takes advantage of the carefree, playful aspects of the child within us to find a space of joy and vibrancy that allows the tension of our adult world to melt away. This technique is quite effective with all headaches, including migraines, which may be caused by or intensified by tension.

If you have a sinus infection, see your doctor. If a pain is telling you to change your environment, deal with it by changing your environment. If you want to see a headache as a reminder of a way to bring more joy into your life, read on.

Presenting Issue:

Good afternoon, Linda. What would you like to work on today?

> "I occasionally get migraine headaches on top of my other issues. They can devastate me for days."

The Dance of Ideas:

Body tensions lead to imbalances and restrictions of blood flow that spiral into full blown headaches. At any time, and certainly the sooner the better, a person can interrupt the process with relaxation. There are specific movements and playful memories that are particularly effective. A memory of running in sun-shine can wash away headache pain.

Practice:

The following induction[9] is contained in several text boxes. As you read the induction, rotate your head in the direction of the arrow in the *Running in Sunshine* box that you are reading. Your head rotation should be much faster than your reading. Try two seconds per rotation and, without count-ing, allow at least three or four rotations as your read each box.

You may have to refocus often and read slowly. That is fine. If you lose your place hold your reading until you find it again on the next (head rota-tion) time around. Take your time and enjoy this exercise.

Please read these directions for the running-in-sunshine headache cure through at least once, so you understand what is coming, then apply them to the boxed induction:

Step 1:   Rotate your head as you slowly read the *Running in Sunshine* box, Breathe often, easily and naturally.

            Take a slow breath and let it out.

Step 2:   Move on to the *More Running in Sunshine* box, reversing the direction of head rotation. As you continue with the exer-cise, a little vertigo is natural and appropriate. This exercise is designed to cure a headache. We will cover curing nausea in a later exercise.

            After you read the text and get a sense of the vision, close your eyes and continue your head rotation as you live the experience in your mind's eye for a minute or two.

            Take a slow breath and let it out.

---

9   This exercise is based in part on a technique I learned from Robert Otto, CHT, at the 2005 ACHE conference in Glendale, CA. Thanks Robert.

Step 3:   Reverse direction again, as you continue with the *Really Running in Sunshine* box.

After you read the text and get a sense of the vision, close your eyes and continue your head rotation as you live the experience in your mind's eye for a minute or two.

Take a slow breath and let it out.

Step 4:   As you get to the "..." at the end of the box, let your head stop moving, your eyes close, and your chin drop to your chest. With eyes closed you may sit back and rest against one of the trees in the field for a few minutes.

Take a slow breath and let it out.

Step 5:   Eventually you return to find yourself sitting with this book in your hand. Welcome back. You have just been to your healing place. Go there when you need a rest. Go there whenever you feel tense.

After returning to this section and performing this exercise a few times, you will find that your healing place is readily available. Can you get to this state quickly by using the finger-drop with intention? Come back later and try it.

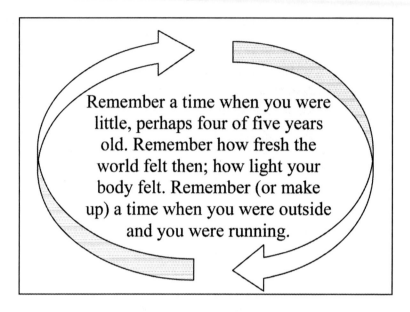

Running in Sunshine

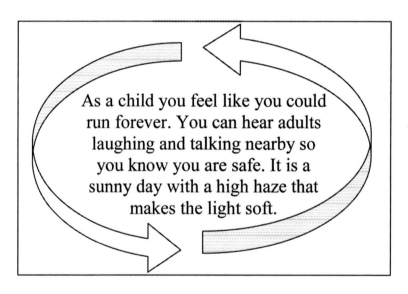

More Running in Sunshine

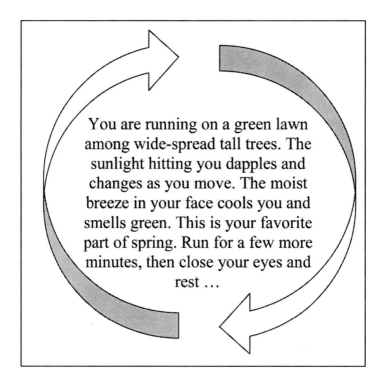

You are running on a green lawn among wide-spread tall trees. The sunlight hitting you dapples and changes as you move. The moist breeze in your face cools you and smells green. This is your favorite part of spring. Run for a few more minutes, then close your eyes and rest ...

Really Running in Sunshine

Homework:

- Practice self-hypnosis.

- Go to your healing place for headache as needed.

- Can you repeat the "Running in Sunshine" three-part exercise and find a joyful giggle somewhere in your experience of your healing place?

- Pay attention to the special shade of purple (or your unique personal signal) when it shows up. Remember, this is you trying to talk with you.

- Recognize pain as a compelling attention getter.

- Be sure to get up, stretch, and perhaps take a walk before reading further.

4.4 IT IS ALL ABOUT ME, ME, ME

Presenting Issue:

Good afternoon, Linda. You look upset. What is going on?

"I feel childish. I want my needs to come first. It is all about me, me, me!"

The Dance of Ideas:

Well of course. You are in pain and you need someone to kiss the boo-boo. Chronic pain wears us out and we need a rest, someone else to care for us. As adults, we cannot count on the unconditional love and attention young children get (or at least should get). As our chronic pain stays with us through the months and years, we will strain even the most loving and unselfish caregivers.

Practice:

Recognize that it is all about you and that is OK. Follow these steps as best you can. The point of this exercise is further integration of the adult you and the child you.

Find a place where you are alone, and are unlikely to be interrupted or overheard. If you have roommates tell them that you are going to work a process for a few minutes that may be loud. You may end up talking to yourself during the following exercise, either silently or out loud; you may also find yourself expressing a lot of emotion, either silently or out loud. Most people do.[10]

I invite you to allow the adult in you to comfort and protect the child. Pick up a teddy bear, a rolled blanket, or a pillow. Hug it to you. Comfort it and cherish it like you would a child. Now picture yourself as that child; accept and relax into that full, comforting embrace.

Now that you have done this consciously, use your finger-drop to allow yourself to drift into trance. Your intention while in trance will be to open your eyes, pick up the surrogate baby (you) and hug it. Close your eyes

---

10 I know that this exercise is not always easy. If you find it difficult please persevere. The rewards of self-integration will be worth it. If it is still too difficult for you, skip it for now. We will revisit the exercise in more detail in a later chapter.

and feel the hugging you receive. Let the comfort you are sending fade into the background as you keep your focus on the comfort you are receiving. Take the time you need to really feel loved. You deserve it. You have had to endure a lot to get to this moment.

I invite you to notice that each time you use your finger-drop you go into trance faster and you seem to go deeper.

4.5   WORKING WITH EARLY WARNING SIGNALS

Let's look at how to work with your early warning signal and provide some additional visualizations to help you achieve and maintain balance.

Presenting Issue:

Hi, Linda. How is it going?

> "I have had moderate success at my practice of self-hypnosis, paying early attention to my world turning purple as a message from my non-conscious mind that I am getting out of balance. I am having great success using my memory of running in breezy sunshine to reduce the number and severity of my migraines.
>
> "I am attempting to achieve balance between my need to stretch my limits (not settle) and knowing when it is time to take a break and rest. I am having trouble communicating this need clearly to myself."

The Dance of Ideas:

Please drop into trance now. What helpful advice can your inner self pass along about your inner communications in every day life?

> "I am sending the messages. They are often still ignored."

Thanks, Linda. Welcome Back.

Remember that the purple color is a message from your non-conscious mind to stop and do what is necessary to regain balance. If this message is not heeded, the usual health/pain systems will follow next. If this happens, realize that the (outer-inner) contract to maintain balance has been broken and remake the contract. Your non-conscious mind is very forgiving. Just keep paying attention and eventually your new desired life-affirming behaviors will fall into place.

Have you come up with any images that can help explain what you are feeling now?

> "I see myself as a trapeze artist. I am safe holding the bar I know about, I am in my comfort zone. I can see the place I want to be as the other trapeze bar comes toward me, but to get to it I have to let go of the bar that I am holding. When I am between bars it is scary and then I need to know that there is a safety net below me to catch me if need be."

The trapeze bars can represent ways of holding who we are (our position) in the world. We know how we dealt with our situation up to now and it must be working because we have survived. Most people have trouble letting go. Even if they can see where they want to be, they do not know how they will actually feel once they get there and they certainly do not know what the transition will be like! Most of us would rather stay in an uncomfortable situation we know about than move to a situation that we do not know about, no matter how positive the change might be! Please drop back into trance and see if you are ready to take on the adventure of change.

> "Life is a mystery. Actions are movement through the unknown. I can drop the illusion that I can hold on to anything, relax, and let myself fall."

Fantastic! We will discuss this further in the future.[11]

4.6   VIGILANCE

Many of us learned early in life to be vigilant; to watch out for the danger in any and every situation. In some cases, perhaps in response to our past traumas, we end up in a state of hyper-vigilance. This section attempts some insight into that situation.

---

11   This theme will be addressed at length in later chapters when we look at the language of the mind and the creation of inner and outer misconceptions.

Presenting Issue:

Good afternoon, Linda. You seem pretty intense today, what is going on for you?

> "Hyper-vigilance does not serve me well. Healthy vigilance is hard to spot.
>
> "I need permission to be, to do things differently. I feel scared of the unknown."

The Dance of Ideas:

It may be useful to change the image that you are currently holding about your situation. What do you have to say in trance?

> "I can move from fear of the unknown to curiosity about the unknown. Then the trapeze net can meet and enfold me rather than my falling into it. So there is no falling and catching, instead there is enfolding and cocooning as my child-like curiosity takes me easily to the next way of being made possible by my ever expanding awareness."

The discussion with Linda gave rise to a diagram of one possible image transformation (Interpret the "→" as "transforms into"):

Fear (Falling to safety)→
 Curiosity (Wrapped in safety) →
  Curiosity welcomes the world!

When we move from a position of viewing the world with fear to a position of viewing the world with curiosity, then change is no longer hard. Life is a grand experiment, and we get to try a change and view the results. It is OK for change to be easy!

As I shared this, Linda had the following epiphany:

> "The insights I have gained over the past sessions do not have to be earth shaking. I am taking things I know and integrating them into new ways of being. The results are earth shaking!"

Practice:

Play with being curious. Try new viewpoints.

Can you read this sentence while you are holding this book upside down?

Can you read the sentence while holding the book up to a mirror?

4.7   COUGHING

Presenting Issue:

Good afternoon, Linda. What's happening?

> "I have been coughing since the last session. What is that about?"

The Dance of Ideas:

I don't know. Please drop into trance and ask yourself. I will record your answer.

> "I am angry! My patience is at an end. I am angry about the way I feel. I am angry about a lot of things I have to do alone. I am angry now that I realize that I placed unreasonable limits on my curiosity. I am tired of doing that! I am not out of control and do not need limits placed on me!"

Linda and I go through an exercise which will be provided to you in a few pages (see Practice) and then I ask. *What insights do you have now?*

> "I can use the anger energy to look forward to what other things I can do to be even more in balance. I do not have to limit myself to just being in balance in the moment. I can be in balance in such a way that it carries into the future."

Linda has not realized it yet, but at this point she has made a fundamental basic shift in her ability to deal with her situation. Through the years of dealing with her suffering she has had plenty of time to go through the stages of grief.[12] Now that she is back in touch with the parts of her that

---

12 The classic five stages of grief, as defined by Elisabeth Kubler-Ross, are: Denial, Anger, Bargaining, Depression, and Acceptance. Passive acceptance

experience anger she has powerful allies in her search for freedom. Anger is a powerful motivator and a powerful pain modifier. In many cases the pain can be modified in the direction of less pain.

I imagine that boxers can do what they do because they effectively use their rage to hit the other guy and to generate the adrenaline that keeps them from feeling the pain from the punishment that they are taking. I believe that although adrenaline is good at pain reduction, endorphins are better, so I invite a person to generate endorphins whenever possible, which is what I did with Linda (see the next paragraph). However, it is nice to know that when I am not in the space to generate endorphins, I can still generate some adrenaline. If I cannot get mellow, at least I can get mad![13]

Linda, I invite you to notice that anger accepted as a gift gives a person energy to apply to life in general and, in this process of acceptance, anger transforms into enthusiasm. Realize that you are not accepting your suffering; you are only accepting your anger about your suffering!

I invite you to consider that there may be an inner way of being in balance that eliminates the need for coughing. This process can proceed on an inner level without conscious involvement. This inner balance is life-supportive and is internally integrated with all of the parts of your personality [both suggestion and Useful Truth]. *I invite you to consider that being in balance is not a task; it is a reward!*

As Linda considered these words her throat relaxed and her breathing evened and deepened. I do not have a good explanation for why holding a positive possibility creates the space for that possibility to manifest, I just notice that sometimes it does.

I also suggested to Linda that she make a point of drinking more water. This experiment has no bad side effects.

---

is useful in situations that we can do nothing about. But this book is about taking charge of the situation that you find yourself in. The goal is freedom, and there is nothing passive about freedom!

13 Adrenaline is the body-produced hormone that stimulates and enables the fight-flight response to danger or injury. Its action includes increased heart rate, changed blood flow, focused awareness, opened airways, and temporary freedom from pain. Endorphins are the class of body-produced hormones associated with pleasure. Their actions include pain reduction and a sense of well being.

Practice:

To uncover the anger part of that last discovery, Linda and I used a pillow to express the anger physically during our session. We looked for a life-affirming way of being with the anger that does not work against our health, and we made the discovery that such a way of being was possible for us.

The pillow technique is given below. Some people have a more intimate relationship with anger than others. If you have already been exposed to the pillow technique and do not find it effective for you, skip ahead to practice 2.

4.7.1 VISCERAL ANGER EXPLORATION

In this exercise, we use a physical expression of anger to allow us to get information about the way we hold anger and how we can make use of that mechanism in ways that serve us. I invite you to experiment with this process. Read through the instructions below to see where we are going, then come back to Step One and try the process.

1. Find a place where you are alone and are unlikely to be interrupted or overheard. If you have roommates tell them that you are going to work a process for a few minutes that may be loud. (Of course, it may just as likely be quiet, but we cannot know that in advance.)

2. Find a fairly firm pillow and place it in your lap. Also place a pen or pencil and paper beside you. (I use a notebook sometimes or a clipboard.)

3. Look for the causes of congestion in your life and assume that there is anger as a gateway. (This is a Useful Truth that gets the exercise moving.)

4. Intend to delve into your anger and as you do so beat the pillow until you get tired of beating it or the anger is replaced with relief. (This step is difficult for many people. If you find it difficult, check out the footnote[14] below.)

---

14 Many people have been taught that it is not OK to feel anger. Accept the Useful Truth that it is part of being human to feel anger; we all do. Society's

5. Take a short rest and read the remaining steps. Then make an attempt to follow them if you choose to do so. There will be a finger-drop signal.

6. Grab onto your pillow and use your intention and your finger-drop to go into trance. Go deep. Start beating (or slapping or poking) the pillow. Drop still deeper into a self-hypnotic trance using your finger-drop signal.

7. While you are beating the pillow express your anger verbally. It is OK to whisper. Only you need to hear what you say. What is the story around your anger at this moment?

8. Pay enough attention to the story to remember the gist of it after the exercise is complete.

9. When you are done beating and talking (or screaming) use your fist-in-the-air to return.

What were you saying? Write down notes about what you said and about what you might have heard in your head.

This is useful information to apply toward helping you to find balance in the future. Thank the parts of you that are willing to hold anger and the parts of you that are willing to express it safely.

4.7.2 VISUAL ANGER EXPLORATION

In this exercise we use a visualization to give ourselves a little distance from our feelings of anger. We use the bigger picture to get information about the way we hold anger and how we can make use of that mechanism in ways that serve us.

---

stricture is about inappropriate expressions of anger. Notice that the pillow will not judge you. You can let it keep being a pillow. We are not trying to right the world's wrongs with this exercise. We are only providing a physical mechanism to let the anger out. There does not have to be any story connected with the anger. Consider it the anger of a pre-verbal baby, no story, just emotion! If you cannot hit the pillow, see if you can slap it. If you cannot slap it, see if you can poke it. If you cannot poke it, skip this exercise and move on to the next.

If you have already performed the pillow exercise above, you already have the information you need about some of the ways anger may be useful to you. Skip this next exercise and move on.

I invite you to experiment with this process. Read through the instructions below to see where we are going, then come back here and try the process.

1. Find a place where you are alone and are unlikely to be interrupted or overheard. If you have roommates tell them that you are going to work a process for a few minutes that may be loud. (Again, it may just as likely be quiet, but we cannot know that in advance.)

2. Pretend that you have available to you a imaginary TV control that allows you full access and view angle capabilities for the pictures in your mind. Also place a real-world pen or pencil and paper beside you. (I use a notebook sometimes or a clipboard.)

3. Look for the causes of congestion in your life and assume that there is anger as a gateway. (This is a Useful Truth that gets the exercise moving.)

4. Remember or create a time when you were angry at someone. Intend to delve into your anger at him/her.

5. Remember or create the situation well enough to feel the anger build within you. Notice how you are directing it at him/her. Notice how he/she is responsible for the anger!

6. Let your visualization become a TV screen. You are watching a very real reality show.

7. Let your emotion build toward rage.

8. Freeze the picture.

9. Use your state-of-the-art mind-controlled TV remote, to pan and zoom around the picture; like the camera does in the dance scene from the Disney 1991 cartoon movie, *Beauty and the Beast*. You can see the person you are angry with, and you can see your own body. You are no longer a participant in the scene in any way. You are a third-party observer. You can move the camera to look at the

scene from different angles. It is even possible to look at the frozen scene through any participant's eyes.

10. Pull the camera out to a full panorama to get the big picture. What about him/her is triggering your anger?

- How is he/she standing or sitting?
- Is he/she near or far from you?
- Zoom in on his/her face. Is there something about his/her expression?
- Look into his/her eyes.
- What do you think his/her emotion is?
- Is he/she even aware of you?

11. What is the back-story—the information that would have been available to you if you had watched the whole movie up to this scene? Can you hear a voice-over describing events that led up to the interaction in the frozen scene?

12. Take a short break and jot down a note or two to remind you of this script that you are watching, frozen in time.

13. Can you, the witness, rewrite the script? Just for variety, can you change the back-story that leads to this moment frozen in time? Perhaps the person who you are angry with is confused and lost? Perhaps they blundered into a situation that they do not understand. Perhaps they are just an idiot, perhaps just a clown. Are they to be laughed at? Pitied? Ignored? Feared? Create some compassion for them. Allow your wisdom and your knowledge of the new script to grant them the gift of your acceptance

14. Get ready to restart the scene from a different viewpoint.

15. Use your intention and your finger-drop to go into trance. Go deep. You, the witness, see that there is an off-camera on-the-spot reporter who holds out a microphone and steps up to the person who you (in the frozen tableau) are angry with. The reporter asks, "What message do you have for us?"

16. Pay attention to their story enough to remember the gist of it after the exercise is complete.

17. When you feel that you have heard enough talking (or screaming) use your fist-in-the-air to return.

What was being said to you? Write down notes about what you might have heard.

This is useful information that may help you to find equanimity in the future. Thank the parts of you that are willing to hold anger and the parts of you that are willing to express it safely.

4.8 ASTHMA

This section relates an anecdote on how just changing my mental attitude about something (an allergen) changed how I physically reacted to it.

Presenting Issue:

I know that I have an allergic reaction that is associated with cats and manifests as an asthma attack. What would happen if I treated this as a psychological issue? I decided to run the experiment.

The Dance of Ideas:

I believe that allergies are the body's reaction to something in the environment that it considers a danger. The allergen is first identified by the hypothalamus. The hypothalamus is the part of the brain that sends chemical messengers throughout the body and somehow (in conjunction with other organs) identifies what the body has to fight as a foreign invader and what can be safely ignored. After the reaction has been established, it may be triggered by any recurring exposure to the allergen.

What came up for me when I used my finger-drop technique was that I was not allergic to cats when I was little, I became allergic to cats around the time I was standing in my front yard wearing only a bathing suit and holding a cat. A curious dog approached. In microseconds, I went from cat in arms to no cat and blood seeping from my arms and chest and forehead. I have avoided cats since that time.

When I visit a house where cats live, usually the cats (having the cat-nature that they do) find that my lack of interest makes me the most interesting person in the room.

I used my finger-drop and my intention to decide that although I do not have to be around them, I think that cats are interesting, fascinating, and lovable. My experience with this change of attitude was that my immediate reaction of discomfort around cats was replaced with no reaction at all. After a few hours, I start to get discomfort and I move out of the cat-filled environment. I would say that my symptoms are 90 percent reduced. Such is the power of mental imaging.

Practice:

Is there something in your life that could benefit from a magic change of attitude?

You might consider using your finger-drop to find out.

Chapter 5 Contents

Chapter 5 Figures

Chapter Five
Relief

5   RELIEF FROM PAIN

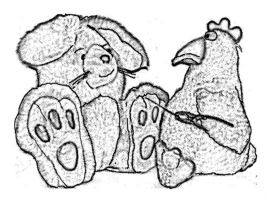

In this chapter we explore our relationship with pain and suffering. We discover how understanding that relationship can provide us with techniques to take charge of our experience. Ultimately this chapter is meant to help you to reach for, and find, stability and balance when you discover yourself in uncomfortable situations that seem beyond your control.

We cover several techniques for pain elimination. You can learn to ignore the pain of a pin stuck in your bottom. This does not mean that you should use the technique to control pain when you sit on a pin. The prudent thing to do would be to stand back up and, if necessary, pull the pin out!

5.1   GIVING ATTITUDE

The techniques introduced here are all based on our ability to modify our attitude as we deal with an experience while still having the experience. These techniques allow us to deal with strong sensations while still noticing that the sensations are there.

Presenting Issue:

Hi, Linda. What would you like to work on today?

> "Now that I have a basic working relationship with my inner self, how can I reduce the level of pain in my life?"

The Dance of Ideas:

I define pain as a strong sensation interpreted through a filter of fear.[15] We know how much it hurts and we are afraid that it will hurt more. We are trying to pull away from the sensation the way we would pull our hand away from a hot stove, but the pain is radiating from a part of our body, so we cannot pull away. As the sensation strengthens and we realize that we are stuck with it, a feeling of fear or even panic can set in. With the onset of the fear, we are in pain and we are suffering. If we can manage the fear we can manage the pain.

In chapter one, we played with the space of joy that comes just before a giggle. In the joy space there is no room for fear and hence no pain. This section suggests other approaches to change our relationship with pain.

One of the things we naturally do when we are trying to get away from a strong sensation is to try to provide a space between it and our self-image. This interpretation of pain as something to be avoided is supported by the way we use language to describe it. We say, "I have pain, I experience pain, I am in pain." We do not say, "I am pain." (Although my wife sometimes informs me that I am a pain!)

There are four attitudinal shifts that take advantage of our natural separation of pain and our self-image. These shifts can immediately reduce or eliminate our pain experience:

1. **Ignore** (Passive): Instead of watching the pain and trying to get away from it. We can simply ignore it. *This eliminates the panic feelings from our experience.*

   This technique is not so easy to practice. Try to not think of an elephant and you find the task nearly impossible. Let your attention drift to the grass under the hot African sun and the elephant wanders away. I find that this works for a short time and then the elephant wanders back and steps on me.

2. **Focus elsewhere** (Active)

---

15 The American Heritage dictionary defines pain as, "An unpleasant sensation, occurring in varying degrees of severity as a consequence of injury, disease, or emotional disorder." This is close to my definition, but my definition gives you a handle on ways to deal with pain.

This approach is similar to the first approach, but we actively seek out something else to focus on. Other current sensations are useful. I know that my right hip is hurting, but what is happening in my left hip? My foot? My butt?

Here the fear evaporates because we are not trapped with our fear. We have other places to go and other feelings to pay attention to. As I cycle around checking out other body parts, I eventually get back to wondering about the location of the pain and, sure enough, there it is. But I am not trapped with it; I just continue on my inner journey checking out happy places in my body.

3. **Honor and accept** (Passive)

We can move toward the sensation rather than away. Become curious about it and explore closely just how it feels. We modify our interpretation of what we are experiencing. Now there is no separation and what was tearing pain is now just strong sensation. As we relax[16] and pay further attention to the strong sensation, it becomes just sensation. We can rest into it and take comfort from it like we would the presence of an old friend. It is not comfortable, but it is familiar. This sometimes works for a while and then I get bored and go on to something else. The approach is usually too passive for me but I find that it works late at night. Often, when I relax into a pain that has been keeping me up, I find that I wake with a start many hours later. Where did the pain go? Where did I go?

4. **Tighten focus** (Active)

Pain takes a little time to be interpreted. How much does it hurt? If we stay on the forefront of experience and do not take the time to analyze, we end up with only unprocessed experience.

How does it feel now? Now? Now? Just keep making the time slices smaller so that there is no analysis because we are on to the next moment of experience. Become fascinated with the pain.

---

16 In the next chapter (in 6.1.1 on page 102) we introduce a technique that combines focus (approach 2) and acceptance (approach 3). There we suggest the possibility of modifying our self-image, increasing the size of the container that holds the pain.

Time slows down and in the moment there is only sensation. This process is shown in the *Tighten the Experience Horizon* box. In this technique, we are simply dropping the interpretation and avoidance part that makes sensation pain.

This is my favorite technique to use at the dentist. I am curious about the feeling and I do not like the numbness that comes with Novocain, so I ask the dentist to use no anesthetic and I busy myself with paying attention.

The time is not pleasant, but it is interesting. This is the technique I used a few months ago when I needed a few stitches for a deep cut on my hand. The doctor did not want to stitch me up without anesthetic until I pointed out to him that his stitching would not hurt me any more than my sticking the knife into my hand had already hurt, and I already knew what that felt like. I do not like pain, but I hate numbness.

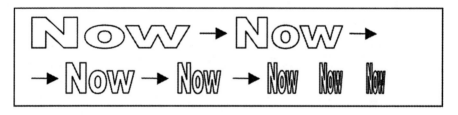

Tightening the Experience Horizon

Practice:

In order to practice pain control, students generally use a clip to pinch a bit of flesh and cause some pain. Then the techniques above can be practiced to verify pain control. Another non-damaging pain test is to put your hand into a bucket of ice water. I generally find that having a person just use a finger and thumb nail from one hand to pinch the skin on the back of the other hand is sufficient to generate enough pain to test the techniques. Since you are reading this book, it is possible that you have enough pain experience at this moment so that you have no problem with finding your own way to test them. (Humor intended!)

I find that, depending on the type of pain and duration of the pain, different techniques work better. I like having an arsenal of techniques. You can rank the pain control effectiveness of each technique for you by using the following table. The pain aspect of the sensation is ranked from one to ten, with one minimal and ten maximal. Read the directions which follow the table.

Action	Pain Level	
	My experience	Your experience
Start pinching to produce pain.	10	10
Ignore the pain for a few moments. Then check back with the sensation. How would you rate the pain level while you were ignoring it?	3	
Release the pinch and re-pinch for a new base level.	10	10
Focus elsewhere for a few moments. Then check back with the sensation. How would you rate the pain level while you were otherwise involved.	2	
Stop and re-pinch for a new base level.	10	10
Honor and relax into the pain for a few moments. Then check back with the sensation. How would you rate the pain level while you were accepting it?	3	
Stop and re-pinch for a new base level.	10	10
Focus and concentrate the pain for a few moments. Make the time slice tight. How fast can you cycle? Then relax back to your normal time sense and check back with the sensation. How would you rate the pain level per time slice?	1	

Ranking Pain Control Techniques

At the start of this exercise you pinch yourself (or get in touch with existing sensation) and notice the sensation. Call that ten. For this exercise, the ten is not considered as the most pain you can imagine, the way you would rate it if a doctor were asking you. It is the level (perhaps relatively minor in your life experience) of the sample pain message you are receiving from the pinch.

I have rated what I felt as I applied these techniques. Fill in the blanks for your own rating.

Which pain control technique seems to work best for you?

5.2   PAIN VALVE

This section provides a powerful visualization that takes advantage of your growing ability with self-hypnosis.

Presenting Issue:

Good afternoon, Linda. What would you like to work on?

> "I have been practicing my finger-drop. I want to learn to apply a self-hypnotic process that I can use rather than the very conscious attitude shifting techniques we discussed last session."

The Dance of Ideas:

Our brain maintains a map of our body[17] and any pain our consciousness experiences must actually be experienced in the map. So the pain experienced by the conscious mind is not the sensation received by the non-conscious mind. There is a gap and we can take advantage of that gap with a visualization practice.

This practice is shown in the *Pain-Valve Visualization* box below.

I picture the nervous system in my body as a root structure with tendrils reaching every place and all joining together in a bundle that leads to a wall map that is set up in my brain. I am sitting back and looking at this wall map. When a part of my body sends a signal, I see a spot light up on the

---

17   Our brains are massive parallel processors that filter and combine sensations to produce what we experience. The part of the brain that interprets experience is located in a different area than the part that receives the experience.

map. The Pain-Valve Visualization provides a highly effective approach to reduce or even eliminate chronic debilitating pain.

Practice:

Find an ache type pain somewhere in your body. If you do not have any, you might consider some vigorous exercise. You can then practice this technique tomorrow.

1. Go into a trance. (Self-induced by Finger Drop).
2. Realize (or remember) that pain is sensation interpreted. This implies an observer (you).
3. Since sensation leads to interpretation there is a connection between the sensation and the observer.
4. Picture the connection as a pipe line between the sensation and the observer (between two distinct locations in your brain).
5. Put a valve in the pipe.
6. Turn the valve toward its closed position to adjust the pain experience level.
7. **Recognize that once learned, the ability to adjust the valve is available at any time.**

Pain-Valve Visualization

I like the idea of sensation flowing in a pipe for this exercise because it keeps the flavor of the pain the same while reducing the intensity. If you like, you can move yourself farther away from the experience, as the observer of the wall map. In that case, you would hold a rheostat, or volume control, and have the ability to dim any bulb that glows too brightly.

5.3   HONOR THE MESSENGER

The previous sections dealt with techniques to address temporary and chronic physical pain. This section addresses the associated mental suffering, the story we tell ourselves about our pain.

Presenting Issue:

Good afternoon, Linda. You look depressed today. What's up?

> "I am tired of being a sick person. I am tired of hurting. I am tired of being me."

The Dance of Ideas:

I like to apply a dynamic variation of the Honor and Accept approach (presented in the previous section). *It is quite effective in quieting my inner voice and taking charge of my mood. This is a method of gaining acceptance of who I am. The method takes acceptance to the level of enthusiasm.* It is a variation of Virginia Satir's "Parts Party" as adapted by the Neural-Linguistic Programming™ (NLP) community. It will be discussed later in this book (section 6.3).

This honoring method is particularly powerful when dealing with mental anguish and the vicissitudes of life and difficult situations, as well as with actual pain. In other words, this technique is helpful in dealing with a person's story about their pain as well as the pain itself.

It is useful to realize that acceptance of full responsibility (in the ownership sense, not the blame sense) for my current situation may or may not help me to move forward toward new ways of being, but denial, rejection and blaming other people for their part in my plight will definitely not help me. Which approach would you like to experiment with?

I personally like to blame others for a while and eventually, when I realize that my approach is not getting me anywhere I want to go, I grudgingly accept responsibility. Knowing where I am allows me to go somewhere else.

Practice:

To start, arbitrarily assume that the pain is a message (this is a Useful Truth!) Further assume that there is a part of your non-conscious self that is responsible for sending the message. Acknowledge that part of you graciously, gratefully, and gladly. Ask that part of you, "What gift, what life-affirming lesson, can I learn from you in this moment?"[18] Now, follow whatever positive thought comes up as good advice.

Many books suggest loving yourself as a starting point. I notice that when I am not in the space of loving myself, I cannot, at that moment, even know what loving myself means, let alone how to get there. However, I always know what loving someone else means. In my case, I have children and grandchildren. I look in their eyes and I know that they are dearer to me than I am to me. I also know, from having dealt with children, with teenagers, and with adults who refuse to grow up, that there are times when you just have to laugh and love! This is the gateway for me; perhaps it will work for you.

When confronted with the silliness of life, either in others or myself, it is always possible to get in touch with the humor in the situation.[19] I assert here, in this book, that if you allow yourself to laugh at yourself, that is sufficient. The love will eventually follow. I find that I like to do this exercise just as I am sitting relaxed. The quiet inner conversation does not seem to require a formal trance. Try it for yourself and see:

With good humor, what life affirming message is available for me right now?

---

18 I know that sometimes "non-life-affirming" messages are available, but their messages tend to be less useful. So ask for the available life-affirming message.

19 If you have trouble seeing the silliness of life, I invite you to stand naked in front of a full-length mirror. That body is what God has created, a hairless ape with a big ego. Is my personality and self-importance any less silly when viewed from the outside? Inside and out, I sometimes feel that I am a collection of bumps, lumps, and bungling chumps. That is why I can relate so well to a Three Stooges or a Laurel and Hardy flick.

If you got a useful message, either write it down for later or act on it immediately. If you did not get what seems to be a useful message, use your finger-drop to take advantage of the trance state. Your intention is to find the good humored, life-affirming message that is underlying your current suffering.

More information on understanding, accepting, and dealing with our self-image will be provided in the sections on the words of our self-talk (Sections 7.2 and 7.4).

5.4   THE FEAR CYCLE

This section looks at the movement away from aliveness that happens when pain experience leads to pain avoidance, which leads to life avoidance.

Presenting Issue:

Good afternoon, Linda. What brings you to me today?

> "My inner child is getting better at play, but the outer me not so much. I hold myself back from participating in many of the activities that are available to me because I am afraid of feeling pain again."

The Dance of Ideas:

I sympathize with you and with everyone who faces this plight. Please tell me more about your experience.

> "After I have been in pain for a long time, I know that any stress can trigger an episode."

I understand. One run in with a bear is all a person needs to be unhappy about bears. People try to avoid pain and stress and in the process they tend to shut down their experience of living. Please continue.

> "The bear is a good example. In this shut down state, it is almost as if I am in a cave hiding in the dark and peering out in fear of the bear's return. The waiting and suffering is made all the worse because I know from past experience that the chronic-pain bear eventually shows up to hurt

me. Chronic pain always returns no matter what temporary measures I take to alleviate it. That is why it is called
chronic. My fear of pain debilitates me, sometimes, more
than the pain would.

"My reading and personal experience have taught me
that human bodies lose resiliency over time when people do
not move enough or stretch enough. I know that I should
practice movement, but my fear of further pain tends to
keep me immobilized.

"I need a way to overcome inertia and overcome fear."

*I propose that since you already know the level of pain that a particular
action will provide, and you know that fear is tied into the pain response and
acts to increase the pain experience; it may be possible for you to just run through
(in your mind's eye) the actions you are avoiding and evaluate the life-affirming benefits of these actions. If the action is good for you and the pain does not
signal further damage, your optimal course is to take action. A life huddling in
fear is not the quality of life I would wish for you.*

*Some people deal with fear by laughing at it. In keeping with the theme of
our sessions, I would propose finding a way to giggle about it.*

Throughout my life, when I have found myself in social situations where
I felt paralyzed and did not know what to do next, I have discovered that
the way that often works best for me is to move in the direction of my fear
and confront it head on. A useful thought is that the emotion of fear is a
"False Expectation Appearing Real." As I actually take the actions I was
afraid of, the fear evaporates and I find myself experiencing freedom and
filled with a giggle. In this process I have enrolled my fear as an ally in my
search for self growth. After sports injuries we all have to figure out what
went wrong, learn from it, and try again. I know that taking action is not
easy, but it is the path to freedom.

Our journey toward a dynamic vibrant way of being requires a balance
between times of rest and times of action. Activity, in line with your doctor's advice, is crucial to continued progress.

Practice:

The goal in this book is to find balance in life and pain is part of that balance.

As in the last section, notice the fear and accept it.

- Thank the part of you that sent the warning.
- Evaluate likely outcomes without emotion.
- Select what seems to be the most life-affirming path.

It seems that joyfully moving forward to action is better than timidly moving forward, which is better than fearfully keeping still. We may have stumbled on another Useful Truth.

5.5   So How About Movement

This session started looking at exercise and ended in celebration.

Presenting Issue:

Good afternoon, Linda. What shall we talk about?

"In the last session we talked about moving away from the state of fear. How do I do that?"

The Dance of Ideas:

What do you have to say in trance?

"Physical movement is crucial to life. I need to move in spite of my pain. I may select my movements to accommodate my situation and my pain, but *I must move.*"

Remember, your vision of Purple (or whatever your unbalance warning signal is) is a notice that things are out of order; it is time to stop and look for balance. I know that when it comes up for me to choose between exercise and rest, I should always, always, always, always consider exercise first. The exercise will make the rest later deeper and better. **Exercise is an excellent gateway to balance** *(Useful Truth).*

When facing her fears Linda had a realization of her own power. She said in wonderment, "It is not scary, it is coming home!"

The following poem appeared when we looked to the silence within us. As I remember, it was a joint creation:

I am my source.
My source bubbles as a wellspring within me.
It is continuous.
I am my source.
I am humbled by it.

Practice:

Continue to strengthen your ability to experience pain-free balance as you demonstrate to your non-conscious mind your commitment to a new way of relating to yourself.

You do this by responding to your warning signal as if it were the pain. I invite you to realize that now you have the ability to have healthy dialogue with your inner non-conscious self. Out of this healthy dialogue, you have alternatives to becoming debilitated. You can experience safety in this dialogue.

5.6   SURGICAL ANESTHESIA

This section discusses the state of no-pain. I have strong feelings about this so bear with me for a few paragraphs while I express them. I will eventually get to the point. You, the reader, might well have a presenting issue by now: "I thought that this book would help me experience no pain, but all you talk about is pain reduction. I want to be pain free!" By the end of this section, you will have an introduction to a set of techniques that can grant your wish.

The Dance of Ideas:

We are striving toward a state of balance, and balance includes both pain and pleasure. There are hypnotic techniques, such as glove anesthesia, that can produce complete loss of feeling. I personally do not like techniques that eliminate all sensation because I want to know when I bang myself, I want to be in touch with the state of my body, so I can, as much as possible, live a long and happy life. The people I know that have experienced nerve damage from trauma or disease have to be extra careful because they are not warned by their body of injuries or infections in a timely manner.

I like to think of life as a train journey. Some of us are here for a few stops and some of us are here for the long haul. We long-haul people will have the chance to experience all manner of scenery, from mountain to forest to plain. Over time, my life will move through times of joy and times of suffering. Given enough time, lots of disasters will have a chance to befall me. If I don't want to experience the bumpy parts of the ride, I may as well get off the train. This discussion about the value of pain has nothing to do with the need to apply anesthesia for short durations and for specific needs.

Childbirth without drugs is considered best for healthy babies, and from my experience with the women in my life, a fairly good approach for moms to attempt. In many surgeries, hypnotic techniques may be used to eliminate or reduce drugs. If you want to fully experience total pain elimination for surgery, I suggest that you consult a hypnotherapist directly and use a surgeon who has had some experience with a patient in the hypnotic state. That stated; you can have a quick experience of glove anesthesia in the boxed exercise that follows, so that you get a sense of what full hypnotic anesthesia is like.

Everyone has had the experience of sleeping in an awkward position for a time and waking up to find an arm or leg asleep because of blocked blood flow. I once was awakened by something cold and dead flopping onto my face. I reached up in fright and pushed it away. It flopped back onto my face slapping me and scaring me further, so I pushed it away still harder. At this point, I felt the tug on my upper arm and woke up enough to realize what was happening.

I had been sleeping with my arm draped up and over my head is such a way that blood flow was restricted. With no blood flow, after a time there was no sensation coming from my hand. I had unknowingly used my left hand to push my right hand away, and my right hand kept flopping back onto my face. In the pain test using a bucket of ice suggested earlier in Section 5.1, **Giving Attitude**, what would happen if you kept your hand in the ice water past the point of pain? Eventually there would be no messages sent from the nerves and no feeling at all in the hand.

Practice:

It is possible for many people to use self-hypnotic techniques to achieve the anesthesia effect without inappropriate sleeping positions or misuse of ice water. I believe that ice water is for sipping, not for bathing.

Read over the steps outlined in the *Glove Anesthesia* box. If you choose to experiment with this technique, use your intention to keep your eyes open during trance so that you can read and follow the instructions as you step through the process. It is useful to know that you can be deeply in trance while your eyes are wide open. This is the underlying phenomena on which hypnotherapists rely when they make post-hypnotic suggestions.

Remember, intend to stay in trance with your eyes open, so you can read and follow the directions.

1. Use your finger-drop to fall into a deep trance.

2. Let your **other hand** rest on a chair arm or a table next to you.

3. Let the resting arm and hand go numb. It is made of grey clay. Notice the tingling feeling in the hand that soon becomes no feeling at all.

4. Use your finger-drop to fall still deeper. It is as if there is virtually no blood flow to your "dead" hand. (As I did this it felt to me as if my arm was missing from the shoulder downward.)

5. Spend a few minutes picturing a bowl of ice water with a hand in it. Just a hand, not your hand. Your hand is on vacation.

6. Use your fist-in-the-air return signal and immediately reach over and pinch the back of your cold, dead (but returning to aliveness) hand. Notice the feeling (or lack of feeling).

7. After you use your return signal to come back to waking consciousness, you will almost immediately have movement back, but it takes a few minutes for the reduced circulation in the test hand resulting from the self-hypnosis to return to normal. The process of going from no-feeling to tingling to full sensation takes a little time.

8. As soon as movement returns, reach over with your recovering hand and pinch the back of your signal hand. Ouch!

Glove Anesthesia

Some folk find this exercise easy and interesting and some experience little effect. Many people, including me, like to stay aware, and anesthesia effectively drops a portion of our awareness. These people may require the active presence of a professional hypnotherapist to stand in for their conscious mind and help them through the exercise. Alternatively, a person may want to make an audio recording of the steps so that they can act as their own hypnotherapist. If you should do this, you can then close your eyes and follow the instructions that you tell yourself.

After you have experimented with reading the "Glove Anesthesia" exercise with intention, stop and make mental note of your experience. You may repeat the exercise to see if the results vary with practice, or just move on to the rest of the book if you have no current interest in anesthesia. This exercise and the support of the hypnotherapist community will be available in the future if you need it.

5.6.1 SELECTIVE BODY PART ANESTHESIA

During a hypnosis session, the hypnotherapist will run through a variation of the glove anesthesia exercise several times and then provide a post-hypnotic suggestion that can trigger the same state of anesthesia. Glove anesthesia may be used as a gateway to anesthesia in any part of the body. The instruction is simply to move the anesthetized hand to the part of your body that you desire to be numbed. Allow the numbness to flow into the desired area. Allow the numbness to grow deeper as you allow yourself to go ever deeper into trance state with each relaxing breath.

There is a fascinating film that was produced by Channel 4 in the UK and was available on the web. It shows a hernia operation live without anesthetic. The patient talks with the doctors during the operation. After the operation he stands up and moves to a chair for recovery.[20] The same hypnotist has produced similar results with multiple patients.

---

20 The patient was hypnotized by London hypnotherapist, John Butler, and the surgery was performed by London surgeon, Tom Hennigan. It was televised live on April 10, 2006. It may still be available for viewing at www.channel4. com.

Chapter 6 Contents

Chapter 6 Figures

Chapter Six
Community

6 BALANCING YOURSELF AND YOUR COMMUNITY

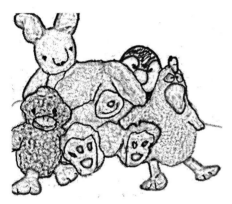

Up to now, we have used our pain experience to drive us deeper into understanding and being with ourselves. We have used it as a motivation to drill into our core. In this chapter, we use it to move in the other direction. We allow the pain to drive us out into the world where we may be of service. The story is no longer about who I am as a body; it becomes about who I am as a community.

6.1 THERE IS LOTS OF "ME" IN "TEAM"

This section considers the individual as part of a social group. It introduces the issues of caregiving, care receiving, and co-dependency that come up during any long illness.

Presenting Issue:

Hello, Linda. What would you like to work on today?

"I need a team to help me. How do I get, honor, acknowledge, and maintain a support group?"

The Dance of Ideas:

Great question! What wisdom does your non-conscious mind have to share on this topic?

> "It is (still) an issue of balance. I accept that giving and receiving for an individual balances out over time. Within the community, the balance between giving and receiving is much more complex. In most cases, individuals are given the opportunity to play both roles within their lifetime.
>
> "My conscious mind has trouble being clear about role participation over time. Quality is also a factor, as is the fact that since I often do not see the whole story, I may be giving when I think I am receiving and visa versa.
>
> "When I think about the life of a community, I get even more confused as to who gives the gift and who receives it. I guess it is an interacting balance of meshing relationships."

Thank you, Linda. I know what you mean.

The Jewish faith defines the concept of "Mitzvah:" A Mitzvah is a duty that in its performance becomes a blessing. At thirteen years old, a child becomes an adult member of the community. A Bar/Bat Mitzvah ceremony is held, during which the person leads the prayers and reads from the Torah in front of the community for the first time. The person becomes a male or female child (bar/bat) of duty/blessing, ready to give and receive in the adult community.

In asking and responding to this issue, Linda has made a quantum leap forward in her relationship with suffering. She is coming out of the shell that her suffering had created around her and is ready to actively reach out and be a part of the greater world. Part of this is acknowledging the people already in her life and part of this is finding new people to share her experience.

It is useful to remember that we humans are social animals. As functioning adults, we need to balance our needs with the needs of others, to determine when to give help and when to ask for help, to overcome the feeling of being useless and the experience of not being productive. All of this takes a village. Since I am alone in my head, I tend to think of myself as an individual. Since I am a social animal, I tend to behave as part of a greater societal organism. My behavior always affects others, either directly or indirectly, so the boundary of where my needs end and the needs of others begin is always blurry.[21]

Sufism is a mystical, dogma-free, study of reality. I once asked a Sufi sage[22] to define a Sufi for me. He responded, "A Sufi is a person who can hold two viewpoints at the same time with equal conviction, his viewpoint and the other guy's."

So how do I distinguish where my boundary is? What part of what I experience in my interaction with others is illusion brought about my own human tendency to misinterpret, misunderstand, and obfuscate?

I know that I need to get help from others and I need to give help to others. I know that when I drop my story to pay attention to my neighbor's story, my life is enriched.

There is really no way to know how much of the shared reality I actually experience the same way as my neighbor does. I do not think a common truth matters as long as our separate realities mesh sufficiently for us to participate in joint activities.

I know that there is a color that we all agree to call red. I also know that different individuals see the color with different intensity. Science can define the color as a specific wavelength in angstroms, but how does that in any way resolve the nuances of experience between my wife and me when we both look at a model wearing a red dress? In this case, perhaps all we can agree on is what to call the color of the dress!

I believe that just as we each have a persistence of vision that allows us to make sense of the many snapshots our eyes take of the world, or turn the frames in a movie into one smooth picture; we have a "persistence of ego" that allows us to take the separate interactions that make up our life with

---

21 The boundary is clearly identifiable physically and, for healthy adults, identifiable emotionally. What is blurry is how much of what I experience of another person is colored by my unconscious fears, desires, or preconceptions.

22 Shamcher Bryn Beorse was a yogi, Sufi, engineer, and economist. When we met in the 70's he was promoting clean energy generation by making use of temperature differentials in the ocean. The process is called OTEC (Ocean Thermal Energy Conversion). There are several web sites that talk about him, his writing, and his legacy.

other people and create a story that ties it all together. I suspect that this persistence of ego insulates and, in many ways, blinds us to the real world.

If I accept that my viewpoint may have a blind spot, I can allow myself to be open to experimenting with different viewpoints that can be less limiting. I can open myself to viewpoints that experience less suffering and more freedom.

Ultimately, I hope to have sufficient control over my experience of reality, that I manifest my world in a new image that elegantly serves me and those around me. The practice that follows provided me with a way to recognize suffering within myself and move beyond it for the greater good.

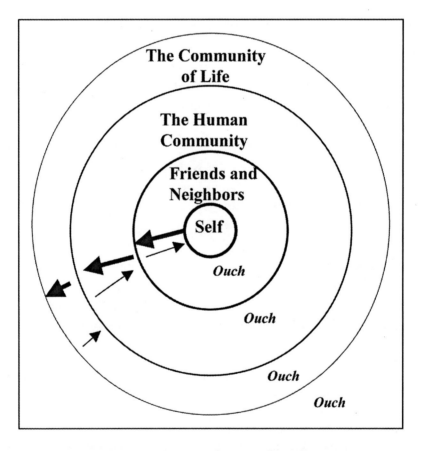

Moving "Ouch-ward" (Outward) and Growing

Practice:

Our goal for now is to access a place of balance and note along the way the feeling of imbalance, so that we can then adjust our life activities as we interact with others to get back in balance as soon as possible. We want to allow ourselves a natural feeling of giving and receiving as the energy of our interactions nurtures us and nurtures those who care for us, or nurtures us and those we care for.

We can use our anguish with our situation to help us grow. Emotional pain means that we have not opened enough. Our desire for community may drive us out of our current (comfortable) circle into the next circle, but after a while our experience of the world's pain may drive us back. The trick is to use the pain to open to the next larger circle rather than retreat. The methods of pain management and intervention identified in the last chapter work just as well on mental pain (anguish, angst, sorrow). Each ring is an "Ouch!" level.

The feeling of anguish is a signal of the loss of balance. We can regain balance by expanding outward to a larger view. The intuitive movement to fold inward stops the pain of the world but leaves us stuck where we were. Moving outward gives us a bigger base upon which we can maintain balance in the future.

If we fold inward what we are really doing is curling in on our fear. If instead, we move outward we may have the same fear but we have a larger area to contain it so our experience is less intense.

As Linda and I studied the diagram in the *Moving "Ouch-ward"* box and experimented with experiencing a bigger concept of who we are, another way of looking at our growth toward freedom occurred to us. Try this visualization: *Suspended and nurtured, floating on the water, I open like a lotus blossom to accept my present level of awareness and expand to the next level. It is not scary, it is home.*

Remember you are not your symptoms! Call it "the illness" rather than "my illness; it is not personal.

6.1.1 Growing Beyond the Edge of Pain

Although the last section applied the "growing-bigger" idea to mental anguish, the technique works just as well for physical pain. In his book *Who Dies?* Stephen Levine[23] provides techniques for relaxing into and thereby softening our resistance to pain sensations.

Levine describes an experiment at the Springrove Clinic in Maryland. Cancer patients in extreme pain were given mild dosages of psychedelics. Those who had a transcendent "one with nature" experience afterward seemed able to maintain a more spacious relationship to themselves. Some who had previously been incapacitated had little or no pain for months afterward. Levine concludes, "… not that the pain had gone away but that the container, the space within which that sensation was experienced, had greatly increased … As the experience of being expands, the experience of pain changes."

6.2 The Play of Programs & Meta-programs

This section distinguishes between what we expect of ourselves and what we think the world expects of us. In NLP terms these two aspects of our belief system are called programs and meta-programs (or behavioral model and behavioral meta-model). They are discussed here because if our programs and meta-programs are not congruent they can be a source of great suffering. The more congruent these two aspects of our belief system are, the easier it is for us to maintain equanimity.

Presenting Issue:

Good afternoon, Linda. I see that you have been working on social issues since last we talked. Do you have any more insights?

> "I cannot seem to live up to what I expect (is expected) of me. My self-judgments and self-doubt can cripple me."

OK, what does your non-conscious mind have to say about this?

> "I am not my expectations. They were imposed on me!"

---

23 Stephen's book is listed in the bibliography.

The Dance of Ideas:

Linda has supplied a fantastic insight. To understand it we need to define some underlying concepts.

A program is a set of behaviors that are designed to produce an expected outcome. Most of what we do as adults is a series of habits that do not require conscious control. Since I know how to type, I need only think the letters with the intention of typing and my fingers move to words on the page in front of me. The spaces between words appear almost as if by magic as my thumb hitting the space bar signals the end of each word. Although we do not usually notice it, the way we think about things is, in itself, a habit, a learned behavior, a program. This level of distinction is usually transparent to us because we rarely think about thinking.

In terms of making judgments about what to do in a given situation, a person's program is the set of rules that they *apply* to set limits on their behavior. The rules define the set of *possible* actions they might take.

Overlaying this is a meta-program, the set of rules they believe everybody (else) in their society knows and lives by. This is a much stricter set of rules. In other words, these are the parental rules that were established before we had a chance to think about them.

Stated still another way, as a child, my program is made up of my parent's rules for me, while my meta-program is made up of my parent's rules for themselves, which they got from their parents, and so on down the generations. These are our society's rules, in many cases consistent with the Ten Commandments.

In terms of making judgments about what to do in a given situation, a person's meta-program is the set of rules that they think they *should apply* to bracket their behavior. These rules define the set of *morally acceptable* actions they might take.

Programs and meta-programs are associated with the many roles we play in life. We have two sets of rules that relate to each activity.

The meta-programs are as powerful in affecting how I relate to others in my circle of acquaintances as my programs are in affecting how I deal with myself. In fact, since I always seem to have time to replay my memories and judge my actions after the fact, my meta-programs greatly affect how I relate to my past me, as if he were another person. They affect how I evaluate what "he" has just done. I ask myself, "Did I write this last paragraph as clearly as I might have?" Since I have a parental injunction to do my best, I hear a critical part of me reply, "I don't think so!" regardless of what the truth might be.

In summary, meta-programs powerfully affect us for better or worse, and they often exist outside of our awareness.

The implications of this in the way our minds are formed are profound:

- Since our programs and our meta-programs were absorbed from the adults and the society around us when we were forming, *the programs are all arbitrary*[24].

- No matter how much I want to believe that I source my actions, I formulate them, at least in part, against the background of my self-image so *my actions are all arbitrary!*

- No matter how much I want to believe that I live in a sane and just society that works best for me and my family, I got this notion from generations past so *my judgments are all arbitrary!*

These statements are both shocking and freeing. If I accept that all the rules that govern who I am, are, to at least some extent, arbitrary, I am free to examine them for usefulness in my current situation, and, possibly change any rule that no longer serves me. What holds me back from making any change is my arbitrary fear of change.

Practice:

I invite you to remember doing something that you knew at the time was a little wrong. Did you feel a guilty pleasure? I feel this way when I take an

---

24 The programs are arbitrary in the sense that they could have been almost any fairly consistent useful set of beliefs; not in the sense that they were created without caring. The world-view of a socialized villager in central Asia is likely be quite different than the world-view of a socialized Londoner, yet each viewpoint is probably to a great extent appropriate for the person involved. Each world-view is a product of the person's unique heritage, language, and underlying cultural myths.

extra piece of chocolate. The tingling we feel is the war between what we allowed ourselves to do, that is, what we found we *could* do, and what we knew was right to do, that is, what we *should* do.

After a politically insensitive remark that has the audience stifling their laughter, Larry the Cable Guy[25] says, "Now you know that that-there was funny." I find myself laughing and feeling bad about it, then laughing even more at myself. Thanks, Larry.

6.3   PARTS PARTY

Earlier, in 5.3 on page 86, I introduced the concept of a parts party. This section expands on the potential for freedom from crippling judgments. The parts party breaks our personality into many sub-personalities in order to identify parts that work together and parts that are in conflict. The idea is to pretend to fragment in order to hear from enough inner voices that all aspects of a problem are represented. It is not that we are really fragmented; it is rather that we are trying to honor different rules for behavior that may be in conflict or even mutually exclusive.

Presenting Issue:

Hi, Linda. The last session was a lot to absorb. Do you have any questions?

> "Yes, is there any way that I can use my sense of commu-
> nity to help my inner process when I am alone?"

The Dance of Ideas:

A person is defined, in large measure, by his or her behaviors. In the previous session, we defined a program as a set of rules that govern behaviors. With this definition in mind, the program that is a person is actually a complex layering of many programs that apply to different situations. Our learned behaviors help us maintain the roles we play in daily life. For me, I am father, husband, worker, playmate all at any one time in any mixture, and all parts not necessarily working as a team. On the inside, however limited my self-perception may be, I am a village. I can treat each part of

---

25   Larry the Cable Guy is the stage name of Daniel Lawrence Whitney, a stand up comedian, actor, and one of the co-stars of the *Blue Collar Comedy Tour*.

me as a separate villager. I can have conversations with the part of me that drives the activities I use to maintain each role.

A subset of this process was suggested in Section 5.3, **Honor the Messenger**, to use as direct pain control. Here I suggest the process as a mechanism for inner reflection and self understanding. In both cases, by seeing the part of me involved in driving my activity as a separate entity within me, I open the possibility of treating this part of me with the respect I would normally give a separate adult individual, of listening attentively to the inner guidance provided by this part of me, and ultimately achieving an integration of all parts of me working together. *I said to myself, "Self, what is going on with you?" And surprisingly, this led to a healthy discussion.*

My sample parts party:

I have a mischievous side that sounds shrill and childish to me when I think thoughts like, "I wonder how upset my wife will be when she realizes X (something embarrassing or uncomfortable). I wonder if she will laugh (not likely)." I try to notice the tone and avoid the game that I know from experience will not end well. It is amazing how long it took me to learn this. How well do you control your mischief?

I invite you to notice your mischievous part, listen to its tone, does it have a name? Is it laughing now?

I seem to also have a voice in my head that suggests loving things I might do. It speaks slowly and sounds reasonable to me. I have learned to not trust it either. The voice suggests actions that I might see as loving, but I find it works better for me if I pay attention to the object of my affection and do what seems loving to him or her rather than what seems loving to me.

I notice that there is:

- A part of me that wants to be liked and gets in the way of my being likeable,

- A part that wants to get attention and might prompt inappropriate actions,

- A part that wants to be seen as wise and gets in the way of actual wisdom.

Lurking under all these roles is a part of me that is authentic and manifests when I least expect it. What is your experience?

Being watchful for the conundrums above allows me to stay aware and be of service to my fellow travelers. The awareness helps me to avoid causing unnecessary suffering for myself and others.

Practice:

Take your time and go easy with these exercises. Try them just a little to get a taste and move on. Note this area to come back to. These exercises may be worth repeating several times over the course of a few weeks or a few months. You may need to use a pencil and paper during the first exercise to help reduce the confusion. The second exercise is guaranteed to drive you crazy. The third exercise will bring you peace.

Exercise 1:

I invite you to find a quiet place and greet some of the different roles (voices, viewpoints) inside you that come into play as you make your way through the world. We are going to have a brief parts party.

It is certainly true for me, and it is quite likely true for you, that some of my parts are currently in conflict with other parts. This is not the time to force resolution of inner conflicts.[26] This is just a time to welcome all parts, be on our good behavior, and enjoy the party.

Think about the voice that is most often with you, the voice that may be sub-vocalizing these words. Does it sound like your speaking voice only

---

26 I believe that the process of inner conflict resolution, other than in the areas of pain and suffering elimination covered by specific exercises in this book, may be addressed best with the help of a professional therapist.

whispering? Does it sound like your mom or dad? Does it sound different depending on what it is saying to you? Get a sense of its usual tone. This voice is going to be the host at this particular parts party. It is the voice that will greet the other guests. It is just going to say, "Hi" to any part that shows up. Let's see who else might show up:

- Is there a part that drives you toward success? Does it have a unique tone? Does it use particular words? Does it have a name?

- Is there a part that blocks you and keeps you from all the success that could be yours? Does it have a unique tone? Does it use particular words? Does it have a name?

- Is there a part that steps up to the plate when someone gets in your face? Does it have a unique tone? Does it use particular words? Does it have a name? Does it say, "Be careful, be meek." Or does it say, "How dare they!"

I invite you to continue your greeting for any other parts that happen to come up for you related to different situations. This is a start on the guest list for this and any later parts parties. Knowing that there is a list is sufficient for now. If you have some time and feel brave, you may consider extending your greeting to a get-to-know-you conversation, or not.

I usually go as far as identifying a part's unique sound and then asking it what it helps me to do, "What is your assigned role or purpose at this time in my life?" When I get a response I do not judge it, I just say, "Thank you for showing up. I know that you are important in my life and that you have helped me to get to this moment. I am grateful to you for your help." I may jot down a note or two to remember the part and its role, then I move on to greet whatever other part might have shown up.

We are not trying to change any part of us during this exercise. We are just acknowledging our inner community and moving toward integration.

Exercise 2:

There is a technique to face and overcome any addiction, e.g., food, drug, alcohol. You notice the voice in your head that is prompting you to take a bite/fix/drink and attempt to reason with it while you do not follow its suggestions. Most folk find that the voice gets shrill and childish as it says things like "Just this time." or "A little won't hurt." or "Who is going to know?" or "I have to have it!" or "You don't understand." The words and the tone are a signal. The technique is then to exaggerate the part of you that is speaking. Make the voice sound cartoon-funny or give it a demon face. Whatever may make you laugh or frighten you. You want to do anything but obey it!

This technique allows you the strength to resist your urges as you recognize them to be the promptings of a child. How hard is it to say "No!" to a two-year-old that you are trying to protect? Exercise the discipline to let the adult part of you stay in charge.

Try the technique now with a piece of chocolate (or some other treat you find hard to resist). For example, take a chocolate kiss, unwrap it, look at it, smell it, think how it will taste. Now throw it in the trash or, if necessary, down the garbage disposal and listen to the voices in your head go crazy:

"You just wasted food!"

"It would have tasted so good!"

"Why are you punishing me?"

"It's only a few calories, what would it hurt?"

"I deserved it and you took it away!"

"You're a *meanie*!"

Notice, laugh, take a drink of water, and move on.

Exercise 3:

In this exercise you identify and personify a part of you that has, up to now, been in charge of prompting a negative behavior. Thank this part for its perseverance and give it a new, life-affirming job. When I use this technique, I end up with a part of me that has a purpose, is happy and fulfilled. To that extent I become less prone to suffering and more capable of vibrant living.

This is a very gentle exercise. The opportunity to practice it comes up when I notice that I seem to be, in some way, off course in my life plan, when my reactions to the people and events around me seem less ideal than I (some part of me) would hope for.

I acknowledge and thank the part of me that has guided me to this moment. I acknowledge and thank the part of me that has noticed that in some way I have gotten off course. I ask the two parts of me to work together to creatively chart and implement a course correction. Then I ask the part of me that is guiding my reactions to consider a course correction and the part of me that noticed the divergence to support it. Both parts now have active positive fulfilling roles in my future improvement.

As the two parts of me continue to work in tandem they effectively become integrated and I become a more congruent, integrated person. If, over time, enough parts of me become happy and fulfilled, surely I, myself, will be become happy and fulfilled. Run the experiment; experience the results.

6.4   ASTHMA

This story from my recent (last few years) past demonstrates how subtle our inner illusions can be. It introduces the concept of victimhood. Do I own my symptoms or do they own me? It provides an example of the self-knowledge and healing than can come from openly sharing our reality with another person. It provides an example of how sharing our reality can allow symptoms and suffering to evaporate.

Presenting Issue:

I have a continuing dance with asthma. (One incident is described in section 4.8 on page 76.) One night at a men's retreat, after an intense day spent working on my relationship to work and money, asthma took the upper hand and I was in discomfort.

The Dance of Ideas:

My friend, Tony, asked me to physically maneuver him in order to see if I could produce the same symptoms in him. I put my arm around him to constrict his chest and had him hold his lips tightened to a small hole while breathing through his mouth to simulate not having enough air. When his breathing got heavy and labored, I was unwilling to continue forcing his suffering even though he was OK with the process.

While we were both suffering the same symptoms, Tony stated, "Assume that asthma is a signal of imbalance and look at the underlying causes." He asked, "What is the underlying driver?"

I experienced an epiphany! There is an imbalance between my story of victimhood and my celebration of existence. It is as if I do not know which part of me to trust. There is a betrayal inside me when I say I will do something and fall short of successful completion. Specifically, at that moment, the time I had spent sitting and processing during the day was not sufficiently balanced by exercise. I resolved to move around and go for a run the next day. My asthma symptoms decreased and eventually disappeared. I popped awake early the next morning. My run, which greeted the brightening morning light, was glorious.

How could I not giggle?

Practice:

There are several parts to the above process:

1. Sharing your state with another person allows you to feel less alone.

2. The very physical process of recreating symptoms allows the other person to gain insight into your situation that you may not have. The questions that they can ask you from this state are often quite profound.

3. The surprise for me was that imbalance was at the heart of my discomfort. That seemed to be in line with the thrust of this book and because of that, it is included here in the pain management chapter.

This practice takes two people, a pencil, and a piece of paper. If you have someone close who is willing to run the experiment with you, fine. If not, skip this exercise for now.

The two people involved are the **giver,** who has symptoms to experience, describe, and give away, and the **receiver,** who has symptoms to receive, simulate, and experience.

Giver: Please know that the receiver is here to help you and does so willingly. Trust that the transaction will ultimately be a gift to him or her.

Receiver: Please know that the giver does not want you to suffer; the pain is reluctantly being shared with you. What you receive is not yours to keep, so do not become attached to it. This transaction is a gift that you are giving to him or her.

Giver: Describe your feelings to the receiver. Where does it hurt? How does it hurt? Describe the symptoms in word pictures. Physically move the receiver or ask him to move into different positions until it looks to you that he is suffering what you are suffering.

Receiver: Follow directions, as best you can, until you feel that you are experiencing the same symptoms as the giver. Pay attention to the feelings that come up for you. When you feel that you and the giver are one, ask the question that comes up for you. Remember, this is not your question, so do not be attached to it any more than you are attached to the symptoms. Having asked the question, your job is done. Step back, relax, and listen. You may want to take notes.

Giver: When you hear the question, intend to answer it and use your finger-drop to drop into a trance. And now, with eyes closed, state whatever answer comes up for you without judgment. Then use your fist-in-the-air to raise yourself back to waking consciousness.

Give this step some time.

Giver and **Receiver** discuss what has been learned.

Chapter 7 Contents

Chapter 7 Figures

Chapter Seven
Self-Talk

7 BALANCING YOUR SELF-TALK

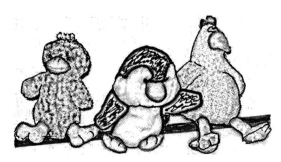

So much of our self-image is tied up with the story that we continually tell ourselves, that it is extremely useful to look at the nature of words, how words affect us in ways we know and how they affect us in ways we probably do not even suspect.

It is interesting to realize that in human communications, roughly 50 percent of the meaning of a message is transmitted by our body language, 40 percent by our tonality, and only 10 percent by the actual meaning of the words.[27] How do those percentages break down in our internal dialogues? In writing this book to communicate with you, I am limited to just the word meanings.

When I realize that in order to communicate, I have to translate the pictures, words, and feelings in my head into characters (which form words and spaces) with my fingers. And then you have to retranslate the patterns of characters back into words and run them through your own processing in order to produce comparable pictures, words, and feelings in your head. I consider it a major miracle if any useful information gets transmitted.

---

27 In *10 Simple Secrets of the World's Greatest Business Communicators,* Carmine Gallo states, "Only a small percentage of communication involves actual words: 7%, to be exact. In fact, 55% of communication is visual (body language, eye contact) and 38% is vocal (pitch, speed, volume, tone of voice)."

7.1 THE INSIDE STORY

The following section deals with how the wording of our thoughts makes us feel.

- Happy thoughts tend to make me feel good about myself and see my roles as life affirming. I find myself smiling as I think them. I want to go and play.

- Sad thoughts tend to make me feel bad about myself. The world seems bleak. I find myself frowning when I think them. I need to go take a nap.

Presenting Issue:

Good afternoon Linda. What seems to be your issue "du jour?"

"I seem to be stuck in my negative (sad) thoughts."

You certainly are not alone. This seems to be many people's experience of their inner life.

The Dance of Ideas:

I notice that, in spite of my best efforts to have my mind be still, thoughts keep drifting through:

- Replays and musings over past events and mistakes
- Favorite joyous memories
- Favorite disasters
- Would-haves, could-haves, and should-haves
- Worry over unrealized consequences
- Worry over the possibilities of unanticipated consequences
- Worry over not worrying enough, and
- Wondering if this list will ever end.

I am sure you have a similar list. The constant chatter swings from positive to negative thoughts and back. Through the use of the technique presented in the next section, I have learned to favor one kind of thought over others. I can choose to spend time indulging in and supporting thoughts that make me feel safe and happy rather than thoughts that make me feel frightened and sad. So can you!

Since the chatter between my ears is of no interest to anybody but me, I might as well structure it in ways that entertain me. If I have no interest in feeling bad, I can focus on thinking a happy thought. If I am enjoying feeling bad, I can be honest with myself and end up enjoying my bad feelings even more. So can you!

I seem to be somewhat of a worrier. On some level I keep revisiting my past mistakes; I tend to be stuck in a "trauma leading to drama" loop. When I notice that this is no longer working for me, it is time to change the script. This does not mean that the trauma is any less real, it is just that I make the story I tell myself about it less compelling. Here is an example:

Story one:

> A few years ago, I was attempting to mountain bike on a rugged trail well beyond my abilities. I was riding down a steep incline and my speed increased past my comfort zone and well into my scare zone. My bike and I reached the bottom of a ravine and started across the rocky bed of a dry creek.
>
> At this moment my rear bike tire wedged between two rocks hard enough to blow out and firm enough to stop the bike from moving. I was immediately treated to a practical lesson in the laws of physics (inertia to be exact) as my body continued to move forward over the unmoving handlebars.
>
> I had a fraction of a second to flex my feet out of the pedal clips and arch my back so my legs would clear the handle bar and not be bruised or broken by the impact. Relieved that I was free of entanglement with the bike, I sailed headfirst toward the boulder strewn ground. I did have another pressing issue coming up.
>
> I needed to protect my body from the impending kiss from mother earth. I attempted a tuck and roll, with first

contact being the back of my helmeted head. The roll went almost as planned, first head then shoulder then back and butt and then over again.

However, as my shoulder hit the ground, I heard the loud crack of a clavicle snapping. I flattened out and slid on my back, accepting road rash rather than risking the next roll over onto what were now broken bones.

When the earth stopped spinning, I was able to get up and use my still working arm to carry my bike back the mile or two to my car. I loaded the bike onto its carrier and drove myself to the nearest emergency room. It took a year or so for my clavicle to stop hurting at night long enough for me to sleep through until morning.

Story two:

A few years ago, I was attempting to mountain bike on a rugged trail well beyond my abilities. I took the inevitable spill and suffered a broken clavicle, one of the most common injuries among bike riders. It took a while to heal and I learned great respect for those participants in the sport who continue to ride in spite of injury.

Both stories are true. Which one has more drama? In the first story I could have added still more drama, blaming the emergency room for the hours I had to wait before I was seen, blaming other riders for not being there to help me even though I had chosen to ride alone, blaming the fates for my pain rather than thanking the fates that I survived to tell the tale. I could go on at length about how dumb I was to risk life and limb or about how selfish and uncaring I was to scare my wife. Or I can choose to tell myself the story with minimal drama and clear my head for more entertaining pursuits, like listening to other people's stories.

Practice:

How happy are the stories you tell yourself? Are you a glass half-full, a glass half-empty, or an I-broke-the-damn-glass type of person? If you had to estimate the percent of the time your thoughts are beating down on you, what would it be? What percent of your thoughts are encouraging and congratulating you for being you? What percent are neutral?

Write down your estimates now. Later I may ask you again to judge how the verbalization techniques are working for you. On a typical day:

Happy/Positive Thought time: _____%

Neutral Thought time: _____%

Sad/Negative Thought time: _____%

In the next section we look at ways to create and keep our self-talk stories more positive.

7.2   EXPOSING INNER/OUTER MISCONCEPTIONS

The same presenting issue prompted two approaches. These are addressed in this section and later in 8.3 on page 150. Here we address not what we are saying so much as the way we are saying it.

Presenting Issue:

Good afternoon, Linda. You look to be in a lot of discomfort today. What are you feeling?

> "My body feels like it is screaming when pain gets too great or is increasing in a way that it will soon be too great to tolerate. Medication is something that I can do myself, while mental adjustment is something I need help with."

Thank you. The way that you described your pain opens up the possibility of revealing some common misconceptions that arise out of the way we all use language in our inner dialogue. Let's consider misconceptions now and look at ways to handle your pain a little later.

The Dance of Ideas:

We all learn language and use it to describe our physical world. We accumulate images from our experiences and use these images to mold our view of the physical world outside us and the mental world within us.

Misconceptions arise because the mental world is not the physical world and different rules apply. For example, we know that the laws of physics impose fairly rigid restrictions on what can happen in the physical world. These rules do not apply to our inner world. Our inner world is not rigid; it is full of contradictions, paradoxes, and even the possibility of doing the impossible.

Some basic differences are sketched out in the table below:

Outer (Physical) World	Inner (Mental) World
Change requires effort. We must overcome inertia to *Start* moving. We must overcome inertia to *Stop* moving.	Change is easy. Thoughts flit in and out and emotions keep moving. It takes effort to maintain the same emotional state.
As children, we want the environment to stay the same. We feel safe with sameness.	We want consistency, but as we gain experience we keep growing and changing.
Any change takes time.	Time is meaningless—there is only now.

Outer and Inner Worlds

These differences in reality result in different appropriate language usage:

Outer: If I give up a part of me I will no longer be me. If I let a part of my body go, who I am will go with it. *If I give up attachment to my arm, I will be armless. I will end up smaller!*

Inner: I can just give up the obstacles associated with a memory, not the memory itself. Fear leaves and the energy remains. I am still myself, only now I have choice in how I feel, react, behave, and manifest in the world! *If I give up attachment to a memory or to a way of looking at the world, I will be able to consider a different way of looking at the world. With the possibility of holding several viewpoints, I will end up bigger!*

I have many times found myself in a situation where my physical needs could be met, but my mental needs might not be, and conversely, I have many times found myself in a situation where my mental needs could be met, but my physical needs might not be.

It is particularly useful for me to notice that there are always these two worlds. But I tend to focus on one or the other and be stuck in it. Integration implies holding simultaneous awareness or at least moving easily between the two.

Linda, please drop into trance and see if any wisdom comes up for you around this issue.

> "As my health improves, my sensitivity to those around me increases. So does my ability to notice and relate to pain in the world outside of me. I see now that if it hurts I need to open more, accept more, flow more, as I find new coping mechanisms for dealing with the new world around the new me."[28]

Thank you. That statement agrees with my experience too.

7.2.1 DANCING WITH A PARTNER

As I look into my past, I notice that I have had some mentors who had good coping skills in one world and some who had good coping skills in the other, but few who seemed to have good coping skills in both. I notice that in my outer world my level of health or illness varies as a function of what I eat, how much I exercise, and my level of physical trauma, disease, and healing. In my inner world, my health seems to be mostly related to how seriously I happen to be taking myself at any moment, what sad thoughts or happy thoughts I happen to be entertaining.

In the outer world I have learned that fire warms but it also burns. I can get close enough for comfort but not too close.

In the inner world I have learned that companionship warms but eventually the loss of a companion hurts, so I tend to keep back from full feeling. Holding back is a mistake in that it keeps me from being fully alive

---

28 Now may be a good time to go back and re-read Section 6.1. Pay particular attention to the *Moving "Ouch-ward" and Growing* box on page 100.

and engaged. It is based on a misunderstanding of inner reality[29]. The truth in my inner world is that if I fully open to a relationship, it never has to end. In the inner world, the relationship is really all about me, not about the other person. I had a very close relationship with my mom, who was a consistently loving and supportive person. When she died I noticed that the major difference in my relationship with her was that I no longer had to pick up the phone to talk with her. I have internalized her sufficiently that she is available to me when I need her advice or comfort. I always know the answer to the question, "What would Mom say?"

I truly love Phoebe, my wife of more than twenty-five years. It was love at first sight. I had the good fortune to meet her just after I had spent some time in an ashram[30] and was at an unusual level of clarity. The best I can describe the experience is that I had developed a loving relationship inside myself. Phoebe stepped into the picture and became the object of that love. Here is an example of inner and outer realities working together. The essence of the love story is about me, not about Phoebe. She is outside while I am inside. I am in touch with both realities and attempt to keep them in balance.

I am thoroughly fascinated with the Phoebe inside my head and joyously think about this Phoebe often. Whenever I get the chance to be with the real Phoebe, I use the time to study her so I can better flesh out the Phoebe in my head. After twenty-five years, I have learned lots and still have lots to learn about her.

I realize that she benefits from being loved by me, but not as much as I benefit from loving her. In like manner, she reports that she loves me. She gets more benefit from her feelings than I get, but I get enough benefit to feel loved and be quite happy about it.

This is a story of balance. I notice that it is easy to get out of balance in a love relationship.

- If the outer person (the other) is more important than the inner representation, then our feelings are not engaged. The person looks

---

29 Refer back to Section 2.4, "Finding the Fiction".

30 An ashram is a Hindu spiritual retreat center. It provides a person with a chance to take a time-out from life. I needed it.

and behaves however they do, but we do not really feel a connection. We may even live with the other person for a while, but eventually we lose interest and our paths part.

- If the inner person (our version of the other) is more important that the actual person, then we are out of touch with shared reality. We may feel quite strongly but our feelings have nothing to do with the other person. Carried to an extreme, this is what a stalker experiences.

Here is an easy thought experiment that helps me stay in a state of equanimity or balance between inner and outer worlds during the ups and downs that happen in a dynamic relationship:

I assume that how I feel about all interactions in the relationship are metaphors for the further unfolding of who I am:

- When I get mad, what button of mine got pushed? I get to discover and own the button.
- When I get pleased, what button of mine got pushed? I get to discover and own the button.

I assume that my partner in the relationship is working on their own issues. I accept that I am a metaphor for him or her:

- Which of my partner's buttons did I press involuntarily? (Or voluntarily; sometimes I like to experiment and test. Bad Alan! What did I hope to gain by that? Did I get the results I expected?)
- The most useful position for me is to honor and respect my partner. The most effective behavior for me consists of those actions that flow out of that position.

I am set up for growth when I realize that any event in my life has the power to change me. At any moment I can surprise myself and joyfully experience a new way of being.

Useful Truth:

In dealing with others I notice that many people seem self-absorbed, self-deluded, and self-righteous.

- **Outer reality**—Relationships with others work better when I give them the space to indulge in these feelings, when I giggle and leave them alone.

- **Inner reality**—I am easier on myself when I give myself the space to experience these feelings, then giggle and look outward.

Useful Truth:

In communication compassion-based (Loving Kindness) honesty is most effective. Surprisingly, this works for internal as well as external communications.

Practice:

You might try to notice any subtle (or gross) misconceptions in your interpretation of your inner and outer voices as they come up.

I invite you to consider the possibility of reacting to each event with a giggle.

7.2.2 CHILD WITHIN

In this subsection, we revisit the child within us and delve into the cycle of love exercise in more detail.

Presenting Issue:

Hello, Linda. How are you doing?

> "My inner child is overextended and does not know what to do. I need to take that part of myself that can watch over others and apply it to comforting myself, to comfort my inner child in all of its crankiness, confusion, and overextension."

Practice:

I call this exercise the love cycle.

What we will do is hug our inner child and send the child love that we, as adults, have for all the world's children. Love returns from the child to us, as all healthy children love the protective adults in their lives. The child's love fills us with more love that we, in turn, send back to the child. We repeat this cycle many times until we feel so loved that we know we are the luckiest and most loved person on the planet. This is non-competitive; there is room for everyone else to feel that they are the most loved person on the planet.

1. Sit comfortably and drop into a deep trance. Use your finger-drop self-hypnosis signal.

2. Hold and comfort the little you (pillow or rolled blanket is useful).

3. Feel your love flow to the child.

4. Feel yourself, as the child, receive and accept the love.

5. Feel yourself, as the child, respect and love the adult that is comforting you.

6. Feel the increased power and self-assurance you get from being the respected adult version of that loved child.

7. From this new position of power and stability, again hold and comfort little you.

8. Repeat the cycle for a time.

9. When you feel complete, use your Fist-in-the-air signal to return to waking consciousness.

10. Say, "I am love."

7.2.3 FINDING AND OWNING MISCONCEPTIONS

I invite you to consider that your experience (view-point) of the world outside you is just a metaphor for the processes going on inside you. This subsection suggests ways to reframe[31] some of the thoughts regarding emotions and some of the concepts that seem to plague our lives. Refer to the table below for suggestions on alternative ways to hold some emotions, then to the next table for new ways one might hold concepts.

---

31 NLP term: to look at a concept from a different point of view, to apply a different framework to the structure of a concept.

Emotion	Frame/Reframe
Frustration	**Frame:** I am often frustrated with the situations I find myself in.
	Reframe: I chose to put myself in frustrating situations. With surprise, "I am open to change."
Love	**Frame:** I want to express my love and my partner backs away.
	Reframe: The most loving thing I can do is to allow someone else the space to act in loving ways toward me.
Humility	**Frame:** I am proud to help others in need, but I do not want my pride to lead me to feel superior to them.
	Reframe: As I help others, I acknowledge that they are helping me.
Righteousness	**Frame:** My version of reality is more accurate and useful than other people's.
	Reframe: It is not about being right because we are all right. We are innately different.
Anger and Fear	**Frame:** My fear of rejection keeps me from expressing my anger.
	Reframe: I can move beyond anger/fear to share my feelings fully/tearfully/joyfully.

Reframing Emotions

Concept	Frame/Reframe
Self-Worth	**Frame:** My worth in the world and my self-worth is related to how I am valued by others and myself. When I feel worthless, I feel hopeless and helpless. **Reframe:** Although it feels hard for me when I am not able to contribute, my worth is not tied to what I can do or not do. It is somehow more related to just being.
Self-Discipline	**Frame:** I am lazy and impulsive. **Reframe:** I can learn to stay focused on goals and control my impulses.
Vigilance	**Frame:** I am afraid of others all the time. I am not safe. **Reframe:** There are some others I can trust. Some people are safer than others.
Compulsion	**Frame:** I must do things a certain way. Bad things will happen if I relax my standards. **Reframe:** I can experiment with new actions and see where they take me.
Dependence	**Frame:** I am afraid that as my illness continues I will be more difficult to live with, less able to contribute. **Reframe:** I am balanced in the flow of giving and receiving. It is always now in terms of how I deal with the world.
Surrender	**Frame:** My fear is that giving in is like giving up. **Reframe:** I surrender not to my circumstances but to my attachment to a role. I can change roles willingly, enthusiastically, and passionately.

Reframing Concepts

In dealing with myself, I notice that when I face my fear of abandonment, anger, frustration, or loss, and I allow the emotion to flow through me, I discover that what used to block me becomes a source of energy for me! I invite you to experiment with this process when a fear arises.

7.3   GOAL SETTING RE-VISITED

When you picked up this book, you had a goal in mind. Hopefully, you wrote down a short goal way back in Chapter 3. This section is designed to clarify parts of that goal in a way that will help you to achieve it. The goal-setting technique that I will describe seems to work in all aspects of my life. Since the theme of this book is pain control and joy creation, I will give examples in that area. Feel free to allow it to help you create movement in any area of your life that you would like to change.

Presenting Issue:

In this case, I asked myself:

> "How can I make use of goal setting techniques to drive me though the creation of this book?"

You may ask yourself:

> "How can I make use of goal setting techniques to drive me toward pain-free, exuberant living?"

The Dance of Ideas:

I define a stated goal as an expression of what already exists in my heart in a way that allows its manifestation in the world. It is possible for that expression to be powerful enough that I feel it pull me to my new reality. When this happens, I have a goal that grabs me.

My experience with the "Goal that Grabs" concept during the years since I presented it at a conference in San Francisco in 1986 is that it is so powerful it scares me. As the goal takes on a life of its own, I am swept along by events and the world conspires to fulfill my dream in spite of my best efforts to fall into old habit patterns that sabotage me. The good side of this conundrum right now is that I find myself writing this text and you get to benefit from what I have discovered. I invite you to run the experiment and discover your power.

The **form** of a goal that grabs has four aspects:

- It is written in present tense.

- It is stated in the positive.

- It is time specific.

- It is activity/place/item specific.

The **content** of a goal that grabs contains three aspects:

- SPIRIT   It moves us toward our higher self.

- OTHER   It involves our relationship with a loved one.

- SELF   It is tied to our own survival.

The goal is written in such a way that it includes its own compelling reason for manifestation.

> *The test of a goal which grabs*
> *is the feeling it creates.*

A Useful Truth is:

> The most important thing about a goal is who we become as we move toward it!

Practice:

The next page contains a sample play-sheet to help you define a set of goals. The symbols are included to help you remember all the aspects of an effectively formatted goal.

The following pages contain a few examples that are in process for me as I am working on this book.

Read my examples to get a feel for what you would like and test their power for you. Then start writing some goals for yourself.

Take your time and expect several rewrites. Remember to test the feelings that are evoked. This goal creation process is lots of fun. When I got to this section, I was really glad that I had decided to write this book.

Goals Which Grab Playsheet

©AWWeiner 1986, 2004, 2007

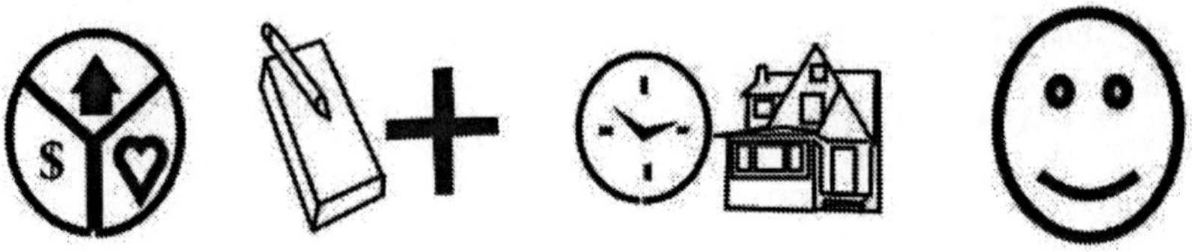

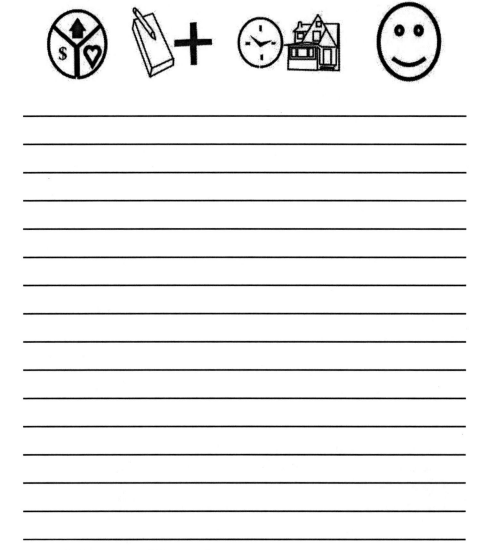

- Include aspects of form and content.
- Re-write until it Grabs—*Test it.*
- Copy and carry—*Read in the AM.*
- Find/draw/make a picture that represents Goal.
- Look at the picture often.

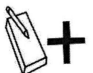 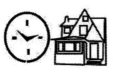

Here are a few Goals that Grab examples, check them against the content, form, and feeling pictures.

1. My wife is ecstatic in May 2007 when this book is completed. It is published soon after with a royalty arrangement that assures our continued prosperity. Reading the book provides many folk with immediately useful information which they apply to replace any suffering in their lives with child-like bliss, freedom, and wonderment.

2. As people read this book and share it with their friends, my circle of influence expands beyond my wildest expectations. Legions of grateful readers thank me and invite me to speaking engagements all around the country and eventually around the world as the knowledge of the joy that comes just before the giggle is spread. My wife and I travel and visit loved ones as we continue to help others.

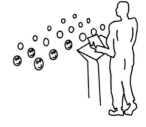

3. From this moment forward, my exuberant good health allows me to engage fully with my life partner and my loved ones; to laugh; to express my love; to gratefully and graciously receive their love; and to be surrendered and at peace while being of service to the world.

Are the pictures representative? Were the aspects of form and content fulfilled? I know how these goals make me feel!

As time permits, make a copy of the Goals Play-sheet page and work on your own goals. Think how you might profit from a tightly focused goals list and how it would serve to help you understand yourself.

Is there some part of your goal that leads you to giggle?

7.4   AFFIRMATIONS

Affirmations are a powerful tool to help us make the attitude changes necessary to realize our goals. I consider affirmations as expressions of our movement toward our goal and celebrations in advance of our reaching our goal. With my definition, when the "Little Engine That Could" says, "I think I can. I think I can." it is not making an affirmation. It would make an affirmation if it said, "I know I can. I know I can!" This session looks at the power of positive suggestions and their effect on the language of our self-talk over time.

Presenting Issue:

Hi, Linda. We have been looking at how our inner language affects our life, shall we continue?

"Yes, are there specific words that will help me improve my self image?"

There are. I suggest the use of affirmations. Let's develop a list. This process is fun. We get to be creative.

The Dance of Ideas:

Affirmations are positive statements presented in the present tense. They express in the best light, what we think or we hope that we are. ***They are statements of being rather than statements of doing!*** The sample list below gives suggested possible affirmations related to mind-body integration and the elimination of pain.

The affirmations regarding pain management presented in the *Suggested Affirmation List* box are depictions of our major life goals in this area. They are similar to a "To Do" list. I like to think of them as a "To Be" or a "To Become" list.

I have love; I am loved, I am love.

Each day I embrace new life-supporting ways to maintain my balance.

My body, mind, and spirit work together in harmony.

My potential for vitality is boundless.

Fear relaxes into curiosity. My safety net surrounds me.

I accept my anger and experience my enthusiasm.

I am whole, I am free, and I fully celebrate myself and the blessing of being.

I am in control and limitless.

I relax easily (anytime).

I am flexible with ease.

I exercise my mind and body as a natural part of each day.

I treat myself and others with loving kindness.

Suggested Affirmation List

The first affirmation regarding self-love is crucial to any affirmation list as it sets the non-conscious mind into a receptive state for the rest of the list.[32] Use the form that resonates with you. You may notice that the list incorporates many of the Useful Truths we have come across on our journey.

Practice:

Many people believe that positive statements like those above which are repeated daily for 30 days or so become part of our self-image. Can you guess what your homework for the next 30 days will be?

---

32 My thanks go to David Gershon and Gail Straub, for this setup to a powerful affirmations list. Their book is listed in the bibliography.

7.4.1 INTRODUCTION TO WRITING AFFIRMATIONS

A positive statement is a statement that is completely free of negation words. Its value has to do with the way our mind forms pictures. If I want a child to be protected from traffic, I do not say, "Do not run into the street!" The only way the child can make sense of this is to picture himself running into the street and then putting a "No Smoking"-like X across the picture. A lot of mental energy goes into producing the picture and just a little mental energy goes into negating it. It is possible that the child will forget the negation before he forgets the picture and I will get exactly the result I do not want.

The positive way to accomplish what I want is to say, "Always stay on the sidewalk." or "Stay away from traffic." or "The curb is a wall for you." All of these produce positive images that match the way the brain stores information. Affirmations are designed to present word pictures to the mind in a way that it can retain and use them.

7.4.2 WRITING YOUR OWN AFFIRMATIONS (1)

A way to quickly create a viable affirmation list is to adapt the *Suggested Affirmation List* presented on page 133 as your own.

Read the affirmation list. How does each affirmation make you feel? Write down the list for yourself so you are not tied to this book.

Use the affirmation list for a few days. Now how does each affirmation make you feel?

Take the time to think about each word. Can you tune the affirmation to be more specific to your situation? A subtle wording change may help you to own it.

7.4.3 WRITING YOUR OWN AFFIRMATIONS (2)

There are organizations that provide weekend workshops that focus on the creation of affirmation lists. This section provides a structure to help you decide on areas of your self image that you would like to modify at this time.

Recall that affirmations are all about the words you use when relating to yourself, the words that define your self image. The exercise that follows is designed to help you get a handle on those words and creatively modify your self-talk in life-affirming ways. You will need a pencil and paper to work this exercise.

Doing this exercise may take some time. The sample affirmation list presented earlier was created and refined over months. I like short exercises so target just a few hours to this effort.

Step 1: What area(s) of my life would I like to improve right now?

Each area will get one or more affirmations. Some possible areas are:

- **Physical Health**, in keeping with the spirit of this book.
- **Mental Heath**, as a natural consequence of a balanced approach to life.
- **Relationship Health**, as a natural consequence of mental health.
- **Financial Health**, what could it hurt?

For now, select one of the above areas or make up an area of your own. You may repeat the following steps for each area you select.

Step 2: What abilities do I possess (or would like to possess) that support this area of my life?

Write down what comes up for you as you consider the question. The list does not have to be exhaustive at this time, nor does it have to contain even the most important abilities. This is your internal list; it does not have to be verified by any evidence from the world at large. It does not have to stand up to any test of truth. It is your inner desire and that is sufficient for now.

At this point, you do not have to be comfortable with your list, or, for that matter, be comfortable with any part of this process. Key to an affirmation are the feelings produced by the mind picture the words create. Eventually we will wordsmith for positive effects, but the creation process is not always pleasant (although it can be). Think of it as a birthing process. The outcome is well worth the effort.

A driven friend recently shared with me that he thinks of his job, "J-O-B" as "Justification-Of-Being." His goal for weekends and after hours is just being.[33] He has an affirmation in this area that helps keep his work life in line with his purpose.

Step 3: Write a statement.

Focus on the improvement area that attracts you the most. Picture how you would be with the changed attributes. Write a positive[34] statement about the new you. Write the statement in the present tense as a declaration of accomplished fact.

Step 4: Tune for feeling.

Add and remove words to both generalize and simplify your statement. This effort is similar to the creation of the goal that grabs, presented earlier. Remember the words are the gateway to the feeling. Strive for feelings of joy, calm, pride, humor, acceptance, serenity, and accomplishment. Refer to the *Suggested Affirmation List* on page 133 to get a feel for how the statements should look.

Step 5: Combine affirmations.

Start a list with a version of the basic affirmation, "I have love." This affirmation provides you with the power to fulfill the rest of your list.

It is time to play and create. If you get stuck at any time use your self-hypnosis finger-drop to go inside and get a little rest and creative information.

---

33 My thanks to Michael Silverton.

34 Positive here means both life-affirming and stated in a way that allows your mind to form a direct picture. For example, an inner-voice positive statement is "Cruciferous vegetables are my friends." While an outer-voice positive statement is "Eat your broccoli!"

7.4.4 Using Affirmations

Use the affirmation list as a morning and/or evening review of who you are and who you are becoming. Read each affirmation (aloud or silently as appropriate) and think about it for a moment. The continuing work is going on in the non-conscious mind and the list is to remind, focus, and strengthen the conscious intent.

Several weeks after starting this process some clients started feeling nausea; we dropped into trance and found an interesting conjecture: "My recent experience of nausea, like pregnancy or going on an anti-depressant regimen, may be caused by my body producing its own set of new anti-depressant endorphins."[35]

In the next weeks, continue to practice opening, listening to your body, and keeping in balance. Your assignment is to find an appropriate outlet for your new-found energy.

I invite you to notice that your vitality has increased substantially since the start of this book and now the issue is channeling and identifying current practical limits. Daily exercise is one facet of a balanced life.

And with that statement, please stop reading, take a deep breath, and go for a walk.

7.4.5 Hypnosis and Affirmations

A major theme around pain control has been the concept of imbalance. Consider adding to your list the open-ended affirmation "When I find myself out of balance, I comfort myself with positive thoughts of ..."

The earliest clue that you might be out of balance is that the thought of imbalance comes up.

There are several ways you might augment your affirmation list and its effectiveness with the use of self-hypnosis:

---

35 My friend Richard Page informs me that, among other things, on their quest for enlightenment Buddhist monks encounter and then renounce nausea.

1. Your goal is to pick up subtle clues to imbalance before the pain shows up. Move your awareness earlier in the process and start making changes before the image of the purple quilt arrives.

2. With the consent of your doctor, consider experimenting with a reduction of your current pharmacological approach to pain management. Please do not unilaterally change your dosage or eliminate prescribed drugs.

3. Self-medication drug dependency can be addressed by realizing that there was a time in your life before there was a drug dependency. Recall a joyous event from that time.[36] Recreate your body-image from how you felt at that time. Hold that sense of self and affirm, "I am drug-free and find it easy to stay this way."

4. Cigarette smoking can be addressed by remembering the time before you became a smoker and how it felt to be that way. Inside you are still that person. Realize this and affirm, "I am a non-smoker"[37] for the next 30 days.

Homework:

Read your affirmations list daily, every morning and night for the next 30 days. Notice the changes in your self-talk.

7.5 EIGHT DAILY ACTIONS

This section is just for fun. The following list resulted from thinking about applying one-word health goals to daily life.

---

36 If the memory of a joyous event does not immediately pop up, just make one up from some movie you saw or book you read.

37 In this case "non-smoker" is a positive image of a person with clean, healthy lungs and a fresh taste in their mouth.

There are at least eight balanced activities that increase the odds of having a good day:

Meditate	Medicate[38]
Ventilate	Ambulate
Hydrate	Urinate
Masticate	Defecate

---

38 This refers to supplements and medication prescribed by a doctor. As we get older, "Remember your meds" is another way husbands and wives say, "I love you!"

Chapter 8 Contents

Chapter 8 Figures

Chapter Eight
Meaning

8 Shared Meaning

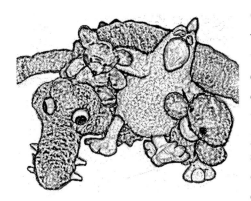

Our self-image is tied up not just with the words we use in our self talk, but also how those words spill over into our interactions with others. This chapter is designed to help the reader experience the power of story. The affirmations and the goals developed in the last chapter begin to be used to change our story in positive ways that can eliminate unnecessary suffering.

8.1 The Subtleties that Underlie Meaning

This section explores how our backgrounds and biases spill over into our understanding of the words we say to others and how we hear the words that come our way.

Presenting Issue:

Good afternoon, Linda. What shall we discuss today?

> "Last weekend I had a very frustrating experience trying to buy paint from a salesperson. I thought I was being clear, but now that I review our interaction, I don't know how much of what I was trying to say actually got through at all.

I think that he was trying to be helpful and I did eventually get the paint I wanted, but I am so frustrated I will not go back to that store."

It seems that you wanted a satisfying buying experience and that the salesperson wanted a satisfied customer. Neither of you got what you wanted although the necessary paint and money exchanged hands.

I have had similar experiences. Even though we can agree on the meaning of the words we use based on the dictionary, each of us adds our own subtleties of meaning based on our unique life experiences.[39] In addition, many people are self-focused and do not take the time to actually experience the impact of their words on other people.

The Dance of Ideas:

We each learn words uniquely and build on our basic knowledge over time to give the words a context that helps us understand them. We easily forget to pay attention to our unique viewpoint, since it is always with us. How conscious is a fish of the water that surrounds it? We do not always appreciate how different the other person's view point may be.

Although each person's pattern of relating to the world is unique, all human patterns are somewhat similar. Since our patterns usually overlap, we are often fooled into believing that a person we are interacting with thinks just like us. Only on the occasions when there is a glaring disconnect do we ask in desperation, "What was he/she/I thinking?"

Several key areas of miscommunication get in our way.

There are gender differences:

I find as a man that I often view myself as being in competition with other men. Often when my friends and I cooperate we seem to be competing to see who is most cooperative. Men feel connected to others by doing some activity with them. This mechanism has nothing to do with language and

---

39 Remember in Chapter 2 we talked about the model of memory formation. The same model explains how we learn words. A word is the label we assign to a chunk of concepts. The specific concepts that make up the chunk are unique for each of us, so the meaning of each word starts with the definition and is amended by our unique interpretation or connotation.

no words need to be spoken for us to feel that we have really gotten close and communicated. Conversation is used to convey information. We tend to take turns talking, or in an argument, may attempt to shout over each other.

On the other hand, I have noticed that conversation gives women a feeling of connection.[40] I grew up watching my mother, her two sisters, and three sister-in-laws engage in marathon conversations. When I was 16, I drove my mother and four of her friends to some function. At one point, I noticed that all five women in the car were talking at the same time. It looked to me like I was the only listener!

In actuality I was not the only listener. The topics intertwined in such a way that it was clear everyone was somehow listening to everyone else, even as their own words were pouring out. The conversation was a joint creation in real-time.

It is my experience that a man and woman can interact and both feel close in activities such as a conversation over dinner. The conversation may be important to the woman, while the eating together is important to the man. He might be just as happy if they ate in silence. This is a basic miscommunication that works out fine, because both parties are getting what they want and may never know that they are each missing the other person's worldview.

There are cultural differences:

Human societies tend to evolve over time from family groups and tribes, to city-state on to country and, for some folk, citizen of the planet. How we see ourselves and the big picture is predicated in a large measure on the Useful Truths or cultural values that we grow up believing in.[41]

---

40 I first learned of this concept is in Deborah Tannin's book, *You Just Don't Understand, Men and Women in Conversation.* Similar concepts are explored by John Grey in *Men are from Mars, Women are from Venus.*

41 There is currently a lot of interest in the study of evolving cultures. Spiral Dynamics, introduced in the 1996 book, *Spiral Dynamics* by Don Beck and Chris Cowan, provides some keys to understanding how our myths define our world views and some of the societal possibilities that may be in store for individuals in the future.

As a second-generation American, I grew up knowing how grateful my grandparents were to be here. I accepted the very American Useful Truth that we gain strength from our differences and our alliance is to America first and our ethnic group and religious affiliation second. I believed that we, as Americans, are powerful as individuals, and, by extension, I believed that everyone in the world is important. In fact, as a Jew, I was taught that to take a life is to destroy a universe.

When the 9/11 disaster happened I found myself grieving for the lost innocent lives, not just American, but all the people who died at the International Trade Center, and all the emergency people who gave their lives in order to save others. In the midst of my grieving, I saw the televised images of Palestinians in the West Bank celebrating by dancing in the streets. I was shocked to my core at my total misunderstanding of their world view. I know now that from a tribal perspective, people with other beliefs are considered as not part of the tribe and are somehow judged as less than human.

I see the same narrow world view in teenagers, where a person is in your clique or not. Many never get into this behavior and most that do eventually outgrow it and become responsible caring adults. There is some evidence and some hope that, given exposure to knowledge, societies will also mature and learn to treat other societies with compassion.

There are generational differences:

Language keeps evolving. We all experience the slang that appears with each generation. In my experience, just in time so that parents have little idea what their teenagers are saying.

There are native language differences:

The Aymara, a group of indigenous people in South America, have a concept of time in their language that places the future physically behind them and the past ahead. In Aymara, "qhipa," which means "back," is used to mean "future," while "nayra" is used for both "front" and "past." For instance, the expression "nayra mara," which is used to mean "last year," can literally be translated to mean "front year," while "qhipa marana," which means "next year," can be translated to mean "back year."[42]

It's not just the linguistic roots that the Aymara have reversed it's also their physical gestures: When Aymara adults speak about the future, they gesture behind them; when they speak about the past, they gesture ahead. The movements seem to suggest that Aymara speakers actually conceive of the past as being physically in front of them and the future behind.

There are geographical or colloquial differences:

When my wife worked at a bank in San Francisco, she had a co-worker who hailed from central Oklahoma and had also spent time in the US Navy. Sometimes when they came out of a meeting that did not go as expected, he would say, "There is a loose cannon on the deck!" She could get a sense of what this seagoing reference meant. Sometimes he would say, "The frog jumped out of the well on that one!" We have no idea what he meant.

There are role related differences:

Based on the situation we find ourselves in, we take on a role and so does the person we are interacting with. We assign ourselves a role to play and we assume a role for the other person. The other person does the same. This is usually done unconsciously. We may be mother or daughter, boss or subordinate, friend or foe. In three-way dramas, we may play persecutor, victim, or enabler.[43]

If our assigned and assumed roles match, the interaction goes much as we might anticipate. When there is a mismatch, such as when an elderly

---

42 I am quoting Rafael Nunez, a cognitive scientist at UC San Diego, and the lead author of a study on the Aymara appearing in the July, 2006 issue of *Cognitive Science*.

43 The Karpman drama triangle is a psychological and social model of human interaction used in Transactional Analysis (TA). The model defines three psychological roles which people often take in a situation:
   - The person who is treated as, or accepts the role of, a *victim*.
   - The person who pressures, coerces or *persecutes* the victim, and
   - The person who intervenes to help the situation or *rescue* the victim.

parent has to be cared for like a child, confusion, misunderstanding and hurt feelings can ensue.

Practice:

Have you ever been wrong as to the basic premise of an exchange, but not realized this until well into the conversation? This is called talking at cross purposes. Essentially two conversations are taking place with neither party realizing it. For a time both parties have a feeling of communicating while, in fact, no communication is taking place.

Have you been happily relating to someone and seeing their similarities to you when something they say brings their differences into sharp focus? A wonderful sketch on the *Saturday Night Live* TV show has three people in a bar sharing personal information. The sharing quickly and hilariously degrades into "too much information."

How is your cultural background useful to you? How does your cultural background get in your way at times?

Here is an experiment you might try. It is designed to increase your level of effective listening. On your next trip to the supermarket, strike up a conversation with the checker. Be aware of her body language. During the exchange, can you notice something about her that shows that she haves a different world view than you do?

A more advanced exercise is to try paying this level of attention to a loved one. This is harder because we care more and may not want to face our basic differences.

8.2   CHOOSING OUR MOOD

This section looks at how our thoughts are an interplay of words and emotions and how we might take conscious control of this interplay to choose our mood.

As the drama plays out, people may suddenly switch roles, or change tactics, and the others involved will often switch unconsciously to match this. For example, the victim turns on the rescuer, or the rescuer switches to persecuting.

Presenting Issue:

Hello, Linda. How are you doing?

> "It seems that sometimes I get depressed and nothing seems to help."

The Dance of Ideas:

I once worked with a client on anger control and together we analyzed our (and, I suspect, every human's) anger mechanism. What we learned can be applied to mitigate any emotional state.

Kicked off by some *event*, our *thought* relates it to a similar previous event in our life and picks up an *emotion*. The *emotion* (chemical release) triggers a corresponding *thought* which gives rise to a corresponding chemical release which we experience as a stronger *emotion*. So our emotion builds until something eventually disrupts the self-generating cycle.

People tend to make use of self-talk as a way to build up and magnify emotional states. Negative processes such as anger can be reinforced by a self-story.

The process for my client, John, goes something like this.

1. Someone cuts in front of him in traffic.

2. He swerves to avoid an accident and experiences the adrenaline surge that results from the near disaster.

3. Heart beating quickly, he tells himself that the motorist acted on purpose. "I was belittled. I feel impotent."

4. His rage builds as his self-talk continues, "How dare he/she treat me this way."

5. His self-image is now threatened. "He/She cannot get away with this!"

6. He brings in an altruistic cover story in the form of a desire to help others, "That driver is a danger to others and that bad-driving behavior must be stopped now."

7. With his justification established, he takes action. He may indulge in name-calling, tailgate, move into the next lane and speed by, cut

back in front of the offending motorist, and make inappropriate hand gestures. This is a series of confrontational and potentially dangerous responses.

Notice how his righteous anger builds with each step in his self-talk story.

Since the story he tells himself is entwined with his emotional state, this opens the possibility that he can use his story to bring about mood changes in a positive direction.

Actually, we can drive our mood in any direction, but it is more fun to drive it positively.

When one of my daughters was 12, she went into a period of teenage depression. She seemed sad and fairly withdrawn. Her mom joked that she was "broken" and sent her to live with me for the summer with instructions that I fix her. When she showed up I certainly missed the bright and happy girl I had seen every summer for the past many years.

I informed her that, "Since I am happy almost all the time I must know something about happiness and I would like you to learn whatever it is that I have discovered. Since I have to go to work every day, we will not have as much time together as I would like. I know that exercise is linked to mood and is necessary for overall good feelings. I suggest that we exercise by running together each morning." Still in the first blush of showing up in California, she agreed to run with me each morning.

The first morning as I tried to wake her, things did not go well. Eventually I herded her out of the house and we managed to limp together once around the local park. Each succeeding day went much as the last. Some days we ran a little, some days we ran a lot, some days we just had lively arguments. She eventually noticed that I really seemed to always be in a good mood and asked about it. "Honey, I am always in a good mood because I am with you. I have the air, the grass, the trees, and your company as reasons, but ultimately, I choose my mood." She said that she could not do that. "Why not?" I asked, "There is nobody there inside your head but you." We ran a few more days.

She said, "I could choose my mood and be happy if you were not making me run with you."

I replied, "That's interesting. If you were to choose to be happy, what percentage of the time would you choose that?" She stated that she would choose to be happy 80 percent of the time.

"OK," I replied. "That works for me. We have twenty days left together this summer. 80 percent gives us 16 happy mornings. Let's only run on the mornings that you choose to be happy. But to be fair to me, since I would like the extra sack time, tell me the night before if its going to be a happy or sad morning so I do not have to get up and dress unnecessarily."

She agreed. Of course, that night she asked me how she could know what her mood the next morning would be. "I do not know, honey, but you are in charge inside your head. Just check inside and tell me what to do." Eventually she said that we would not run. The next night, after a similar discussion, she decided to run. The next morning we had a wonderful time. That night she chose happy without fuss, and again we had a great morning run together. In fact we continued this way for the remaining days. She chose to be happy every morning and I did not get my morning sleep-ins.

Our last conversation on the topic was to address her fear that she had been broken and now was fixed. She did not really want to admit that Mom and Dad might have been right about something. I apologized for our using the "broken/fixed" wording. Her mom and I were having a little fun at her expense. I clarified as follows, "It was not a matter of broken and fixed. It was a matter of your learning how to master your emotions. I provided a model for you, but you did the learning. Your body is going through chemical disruptions as part of growing up, you have mastered how to ride out those disruptions and still choose your moods. Great job!"

Practice:

Here is a chance to tell a happy story from your own life. (5 minute time limit)

1. Just notice how you feel in this moment.

2. Start the story. "I am so happy that I ... (talk about something positive in your life). Not only that, I am happy that I (more positive stuff). In fact, it is amazing that ...

3. Notice how you feel now.

8.3   Using the Placebo Effect

The same presenting issue prompted two approaches. The effect of the particular words we use in our story and the misconceptions that can arise was addressed in 7.2 page 119. This section looks more at the beneficial effects of the chemistry associated with the concepts that form our thoughts.

Presenting Issue:

Good afternoon, Linda. You look to be in a lot of discomfort today. What are you feeling?

> "My body feels like it is screaming when pain gets too great or is increasing in a way that it will soon be too great to tolerate. Medication is something that I can do myself, while mental adjustment is something I need help with."

Thank you. The way that you described your pain revealed common misconceptions that arise out of the way we all use language in our inner dialogue. Now let's consider ways to handle your pain.

Thoughts can produce chemicals which create or recreate a state of mind. My mind/brain/body can recreate or regenerate any state I have experienced, so taking a medication is an opportunity to experience a useful state that (perhaps) I can later learn to create on my own.

The Dance of Ideas:

The approach I am suggesting here is known as the placebo effect, where taking a medication with the expectation of a result produces the anticipated result even if the medication contains no active ingredients.

Some of my clients have reported taking a medication that should take effect in fifteen minutes and then feeling immediate relief, perhaps because they know that relief is coming.

Practice:

This suggested practice cannot be scheduled. Just take advantage of the opportunity when it comes up.

1. Notice how you feel before you take your medication.

2. Take the medication and look for any immediate results. (How much of the placebo effect are you currently taking advantage of?)

3. Wait for the medication to kick in.

4. Consciously take a full inventory of your current state. You might want to take notes.

   a. Get an overall body sense. How does your body feel from head to foot?

   b. Specifically describe your current pain issue. Is the pain experience now dull, now numb, or now gone? Do you still experience the pain but just don't seem to care about it?

5. Assign a keyword/picture signal[44] as a label for this state and include it in your notes. (For example, I think "Mellow Yellow" while hearing the Donovan song and seeing yellow around me.)

6. The next time you notice that you are in a pain-increasing state, recall your keyword and attempt to re-create the state independent of the medication. Take your time.

7. After a while notice your level of success. As a Useful Truth, allow the level of success to continue to improve with practice.

8.4 TELLING STORIES—THE POWER OF WORDS

The issues addressed in this section came about while Linda was relating a wonderful story of her progress in being physically active. She chose to continue playing with her grandchild rather than calling a halt and resting. As she told the story, Linda's self-judgments regarding her commitment to take care of herself surfaced, and her mood and demeanor changed from celebration to self-accusation.

Presenting Issue:

Good afternoon, Linda. How is your inner dialogue going?

---

44 This is an NLP anchor. The technique is discussed further in Section 10.2.

"Now that I am able to be physically active, I find that when I have pushed myself too far, I end up thinking, 'I should have …' and the should-haves, would-haves, and could-haves drop me into depression. It seems that even when I am reporting on a good thing, the way I express it can negatively affect my mood."

The Dance of Ideas:

As our health gets better, our abilities improve and what we can do changes. It is natural to stretch and explore new areas. Sometimes we may overextend. Just continue exploring new ways of being, even though it is hard to be patient with the process now that you are feeling so much better.

Amazingly, our stories can be used to pull us out of the past and toward a bright future. They can hold us back or catapult us forward. I cannot be sure of how my words will be received since I can never know my partners on this planet as well as I would like. I have used stories about my life and borrowed stories from the lives of my clients as ways of illustrating points and communicating ideas.

Here are a few stories for your enjoyment.

8.4.1 BLISS

Join me in a blissful moment:

This morning, I sit here on my couch writing this while sipping tea and watching the dawn break. The sky lightens and the sun begins to highlight the tops of the trees that surround the pool in my backyard. It is almost time to ride my bike to the community lap pool and get a start on yet another day in paradise. Later, I will start the coffee for Phoebe and see if she is interested in sharing breakfast.

Oops, I have to let Max, the dog, outside. He just burrowed his snout under me to get my attention. At 12 years old and 120 pounds, he mostly lies around looking like a large furry rug, but he can still run with me if I go easy on him, and his woof is still as loud and full as it ever was.

8.4.2 LAUGHTER

Energized and ready for some exercise? How about a little laughter?

Jun-Jun, our 2-year-old grandson is visiting. It is the end of a long day of playing together. Jun-Jun's first word was "fish." He has since expanded his vocabulary to include, "My fish!" "More fish!" and "Where da fish?" Knowing his predilection, Phoebe bought several plastic fish and scattered them around the house. One looks like Nemo, from the Disney movie. Jun-Jun immediately claimed the fish and has been carrying them around the house and sleeping with them for the past four days.

It is 9 PM, bedtime, and Phoebe and I are settling down on the couch for some TV together. A little head that is mostly dark, mischievous eyes peeks around the corner from the bedroom hallway. Jun-Jun hunches down and sneaks by the TV directly in front of us. We know from the stealth of his steps and the set of his back that he expects us to stop him and send him back to bed at any moment.

He makes it past the TV and to within reach of the dinner table. Suddenly he leaps to the table and grabs Nemo, who has been resting near the table edge since supper. In a blink, Jun-Jun turns and rushes back past us and to bed, leaving a blur of motion, a breeze of air, and an echoing giggle floating behind him.

8.4.3 ECSTASY

A story can be made more powerful by taking advantage of your ability to remember and re-create your past. Join me in recalling ecstasy.

Remember (or make up) a time when you were three or four years old ... You are drawing with crayons in a coloring book. You have experimented with a few colors and now you are using your favorite. What color crayon are you using? You have just learned about borders and how to stay within the lines. You are proudly and carefully exercising your hard won ability to shade. Notice the vividness of the area you have just colored.

Now you look up and see your mommy watching you. You see the pride and joy in her eyes as she looks at you. Suddenly and unexpectedly, your world expands to include her and her love for you. Your pride in yourself and her pride in you seem to get intermingled. Your love and her love combine. Welcome to ecstasy, an emotion at the border of individual experience.

8.4.4 Blessing

Here is a gift with pictures.

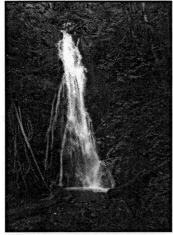

Reflecting by a waterfall:

The smell and sound of falling water, a breeze through the trees rustles leaves and bathes you in dappled sunlight.

Exploring and learning:

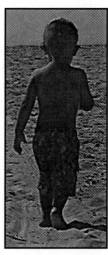

The salt smell, the hot sun, the cold sea, the wonder of love, you shiver with anticipation of the thrill and the shrieks that will greet the next wave.

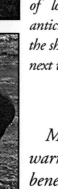

May the ground be warm and comforting beneath your feet.

8.5 No Story

Up to now in this chapter, I have focused on the words of our story, since the words contain the context we wish to communicate to ourselves and others. But the words are not the only content we possess. Sometimes we can dwell in inner silence.

There is an anecdote about an old farmer sitting on his porch and whittling. When asked what he is doing, he replies, "Sometimes ah sets and thinks and other times ah just sets!" In the previous section:

- The first picture showed being and sharing; experiencing a waterfall without words,

- The second showed playing, loving and wonderment without words, and

- The last showed a young child striding purposefully into his future.

Our minds can go from picture to emotion and from emotion to picture without words. Actions can be prompted by a vision and the story can come later.

Humans have other ways of thinking beside the voices in our heads. Among them, we have the pictures in our mind's eye, we have the feelings in our heart, and we have the sense of self in our body image.[45] These ways of thinking are called *thinking modalities*. Some of the different ways our thoughts and emotions might interact are pictured in the *Play of Thought and Emotion* box.

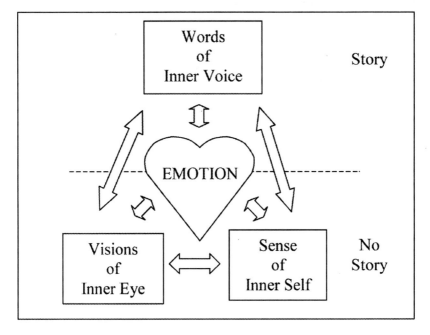

Play of Thought and Emotion

---

45 Alternative ways of remembering and ways of thinking are addressed in more detail in the next chapter.

Emotions and thoughts can build to result in action using any of the modalities and the modalities can cycle among themselves and spiral upward to produce action as discussed in Section 8.2, **Choosing Our Mood**.

Habits are stored in a brain mechanism called procedural memory. I can type without thinking about the process, so I can just focus on the words. Typing is a good habit in that it aids me in the world. Overeating is a bad habit in that it negatively affects my health and longevity. My pursuit of the stuffed tummy feeling may not be conscious until I find myself stuffed and think, "Oh yeah, here I am again!"

Habitual actions can seem to happen without a set-up precipitating thought. A cigarette smoker becomes aware of a cigarette just before she lights it. Earlier this evening, I had decided to eat only half of my tuna sandwich and a few minutes later noticed the first bite of the second half in my mouth.

Practice:

Look up from this book, breathe in and let it out.

Take in your surroundings.

Take a moment to just be here.

Notice what you are experiencing.

Notice how you feel about what you are experiencing.

Breathe in and let it out.

Hang out in silence for a moment.

Welcome home.

8.5.1 LIVING WITHOUT A STORY

It is important to make a distinction between the stories that I carry from my past and my unfolding story now.

The stories about my life have some aspects that may make them less than useful to me:

- Stories are distracting. They get between me and my experience of the moment.

- Stories always have a fiction in them. I can only create them from my own viewpoint and I never have all the facts.

Am I capable of living my life without a story? Can I just be committed to the flow of the day?

I have a friend who is in his eighties and is consciously attempting to live his very productive life without a story. He is a sculptor so he is aided in this by his passion, living in a world of shapes and textures. This is not to say he cannot deal with the world of words. He is a published author.

I learned about his efforts as, after much prodding, he relayed to a group his no-story story. It is a spiritual discipline that has the potential to bring great peace. He attempts to experience the here-now directly and consistently without self talk. I was lucky to be a witness to his success. Since he holds few words about himself, his sharing about himself is brief. He talks about his passion, not about himself.

I found that he had much to share. I experienced his sharing the moment I was in his presence. However, I needed words to help myself understand what was happening. I needed words to pass along to you the concept and the possibility of living a life without a story.

If some folk can live without a story, how free am I to live any story I choose?

8.5.2 A Final Word on Words

I have a friend[46] who runs retreats for troubled teens and their families. He provides an energizing statement that allows folk to stop the useless process of blaming each other and society for their ills:

You always get the results you intended.

All else is reasons, excuses, or stories.

This statement has nothing to do with what happens to us. It is about our choice of response to what happens to us.

---

46 My thanks to Dan Hester for this very powerful Useful Truth.

Chapter 9 Contents

Chapter 9 Figures

Chapter Nine
Emotions

9 BALANCING EMOTIONS

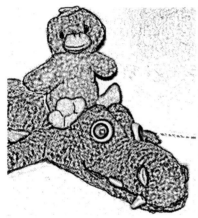

The *Play of Thought and Emotion* box at the end of the last chapter points out the basic nature of human beings. Although we *think* of ourselves as *thinking* beings we somehow *feel* that deep down, under layers of denial for some, under blankets of acceptance for others, we are *feeling* beings. Our emotions drive us and control most of what happens in our bodies through chemical messengers and the autonomic nervous system.[47]

This chapter addresses emotional issues and provides techniques to deal directly with our underlying emotional nature.

9.1 FOLLOW THE FEELINGS

When I see a client I am quite often presented with a compelling story and a lot of words. To the extent that we (the client and I) allow ourselves to

---

47 Candace Pert writes in *Molecules of Emotion* that we can get habituated to particular emotions which create a chemical addiction in our bodies. Frederic Luskin's Forgiveness Project at Stanford University looked at how stress mechanisms that are designed to protect our bodies in the short-term can be abused by our long-term reactions to our environment and result in body damage. As implied by the project name, techniques to help mitigate the damage were explored.

follow the words and look for the hidden meanings and shadings of mean-ing, we spend much of our time misdirected.

If, instead, I uncover and address the underlying feelings that give rise to the story, and if together we can relate these feelings to both recent and his-torical events and actions in the client's life, a pattern usually presents itself. We experience a sense of truth, and the client's unconscious mind quickly provides realizations that expose what misconceptions have been blocking progress. We can then explore ways of looking at the world that will allow the client to move forward toward his or her goal.

Presenting Issue:

Good afternoon, Linda. What are you feeling today?

"I find that I have stopped reading my affirmation list. Why is that?

"The affirmation, 'I support and comfort myself ... I am at peace with myself' is particularly bothersome to me."[48]

The Dance of Ideas:

I wonder why that is, Linda? Please tell me more about what is going on for you.

"I feel totally helpless. Today was a day for practicing cop-ing with feeling bad! It was a day when I really needed sup-port. Today I took on the job of just taking care of myself and I am not happy with the result. This is a bummer!"

It certainly is. Please use your finger-drop and answer this question from your trance state. "What is going on for you?"

"I am loved. I am taken care of. This experience is all part of the process of taking care of me. I am part of the team that is taking care of me, but it is not a one-person team any more.

"I have many more options than I ever realized!

---

48 Because of the information uncovered in this session, Linda and I went back and reviewed our affirmation list. In the list the troubling affirmation was eliminated and replaced by, "I accept my anger and experience my enthusi-asm." Our final list is included as an example in an earlier chapter.

"My inner child is angry. Even though we are not always good at it, we have always strived to work together, but this is now and this is hard! We are tired of wishing it will all work out."

What is going on here? What is the dread? What can we do to help?

"It is about trust, it is about letting go, it is about being willing to walk in the unknown. To go forward, I need to be willing to experience the discomfort and uncertainty of this moment."

Practice:

Review your affirmation list in the light of the above discussion. Remember that, as feeling beings, emotions underlie much of what we do.

Read each affirmation and decide how it makes you feel (positive = comfortable, negative = uncomfortable):

- If you feel positive about it leave it alone.
- If you feel negative about it, you may consider a re-wording.
- If you feel neutral about it, you may consider removing it from the list. In your consideration:
  o If you feel positive or neutral about removing it, then do so.
  o If you feel uncomfortable removing it, leave it in for now.

For the affirmations that would benefit from a re-wording, ask yourself, "What underlying situation is the affirmation designed to deal with, and what is the overriding emotion that I associate with that situation?" For each of these affirmations:

1. If an answer does not immediately pop up, use your finger-drop to help the process along.
2. Write the answers down without judging them.
3. Take a short break.
4. Review what you have written.
5. Use your insights to tune your list.

For Linda the emotions of anger or frustration lead to fear, which leads to anxiety, discomfort, and pain. One affirmation that helped was, "My safety net surrounds me. I feel supported and comforted." One might consider adding trust and faith to this comfort aphorism.

Here are a few Useful Truths:

- Wisdom is the balance of innocence and knowledge, or alternatively.
- Wisdom is the balance of emotion and reason.
- Balance can involve surprise and the unexpected. This Useful Truth allows for the possibility that a surprise that throws us out of balance can result in our naturally landing in a new state of balance.

9.2   THE WOUNDED CHILD

This section looks at the effects of emotional healing on our internal landscape.

Presenting Issue:

Hi, Linda. What are you feeling today?

> "I feel that the child version of me inside my mind is wounded. How can I heal the wounds?"

The Dance of Ideas:

I suggest that a positive action to take is to use our affirmation list to start and maintain an inner healing process. I have found that over time my wounded adult has healed. I can now send love and healing energy back in time to my wounded child. Remember, inside our heads all events happen at the same time and there is only now. The non-conscious mind has no sense of chronology.

We can create a cyclic healing process. The child within was wounded because events occurred beyond its child-like understanding, The caring adult within sends love and understanding to the child within. The accepted child within is strengthened by the healing acceptance and grows up to become an even more compassionate and self-accepting adult. This more powerful and self-assured adult is free to repeat the process of loving and understanding the child.

Although this cyclic healing process can happen quite quickly, my experience is that I seem to heal somewhat slowly over time. I have discovered that there is a shortcut that speeds the process, should I choose to use it:

One pathway to freedom leads through surrender.

Practice:

I invite you to join me in my surrender process. Read the words and own them.

- I renounce blame. Stuff happens. That is life.
- I renounce holding emotions that are no longer serving me in positive ways.
- I renounce holding positions that do not support who I want to be in the world.
- In favor of being alive and effective, I renounce being right!

This surrender frees me and leads me to:

- I accept full responsibility for the world I co-created.
- I find myself holding joy, love, and gratitude.
- I find myself giving care and comfort to myself and those around me.
- I am vibrantly alive and totally free to be in the moment.

Ah, I quite enjoyed that exercise. I feel energized and ready to move on.[49]

9.3 THE WOUNDED ADULT

This section looks at the effects of emotional healing on our external landscape, how we interact with other people.

Presenting Issue:

Hi, Linda. You seem distracted. How are you feeling today?

---

49 My thanks to Sally Clark, MFT, for suggesting this exercise.

"Sometimes it seems to me that everyone I talk to has their own agenda. They are not even listening to me or honoring my advice. This really frustrates and immobilizes me."

I suggest that the way out of this dilemma is to surrender.

The Dance of Ideas:

No matter how a person might feel about what they are attempting or hope to gain from an interaction, it is possible that their motives may not be as pure they would hope they are. I know people who seem to want to control other people's life in some way. With the exception of protecting children or adults whose competence has been proven questionable, this attempt at control is uncalled for and usually ineffective. If the desire to help springs from wanting the recipient to be dependent on the helper, or to owe the helper something, then the helper is best served by giving this desire up.

This does not mean that we have to be quiet, even when we are unclear as to our motives. We do not have to give up our desire to be useful and have impact in the world. We just have to realize that when we attempt to influence others, we need to balance our wish to change them against their right to stay the same.

It is also useful to remember that if someone wants to set us up in a role so that they can work out their own issues, they will do so. We do not have to play along with their fantasy, nor, in a healthy relationship, do we particularly have to be affected by it!

I believe that in healthy relationships, any role assignments are consciously or unconsciously negotiated and subject to change as appropriate. If partnership roles are established unconsciously and neither partner has an issue, there is no problem. If conditions change and one partner starts feeling resentment, it is time for a new negotiation. The feeling of resentment is a good early warning signal of imbalance in the relationship.

This information comes up here because this is the chapter about feelings and communications. When I interact with others that I care about, I certainly have chances to experience hurt feelings. During the hurt, I forget that I also have chances to experience feelings of closeness.

Practice:

Ask the people close to you if they are feeling used or unappreciated. Is there anything that you can do to make their lives easier?

Notice if you are feeling used or unappreciated. Is there anything that you can ask for that will make your life easier?

This exercise is not about actual fairness or about keeping score. It is more about the feeling of being in a balanced relationship. A balanced relationship can be a lot of fun. It is OK to giggle.

9.4   EXPECTATIONS VERSUS EXPECTANCY

This section uncovers an easy to understand and easy to use key to equanimity. The practice presented is designed to relieve the negative aspects of the pressure created by expectations. If a person has no expectations placed on them by themselves or others, there is no pressure to relieve.

Presenting Issue:

Good afternoon, Linda. How is my favorite driven person today?

"I never seem to be satisfied with my progress."

You are being pretty hard on yourself. Perhaps this Useful Truth will be of some benefit.

The Dance of Ideas:

There is a tremendous difference between having expectations and being in a state of expectancy. Expectations are anticipated results that we put on the world and that we think (with some justification) the world puts on us. This sets us up for bad feelings:

- If we fall short of the results we anticipated, we fail, we get an "F".

- If we achieve the results, the best we can get is a "C" for "Adequate performance."

A state of expectancy is: "I do not know what will happen, but I know that I will be pleasantly surprised."

- No matter what happens, we get an "A"!

This path to freedom assumes that you believe that you are trying your best and addresses your relationship with the results you experience:

- Expectations put on me by others are their problem.

- Expectations that I put on myself are bogus. I already know that I am trying (trying not necessarily doing) my best.

- Expectations I put on others get in the way of my experience of love for them. I renounce those expectations and grant those around me the freedom to behave any way they choose to behave. If they behave in ways hurtful to themselves or others, I may want to bring this to their attention or rethink the relationship.

- If I think I want something from someone else, I should be sure in advance that they are willing and able to provide it to me. Remember the old adage, "You cannot get milk at the hardware store."

- I accept my past and all its inconsistencies.

Practice:

I invite you to realize: Any expectation, however useful, has the potential to be deadening to your experience of life.

Spend a little time on something that needs doing. What can you do today that will give you a sense of accomplishment? Notice that this is a *doing* assignment. In other sections I have suggested *being* assignments. Our path to freedom moves through a balance between doing and being.

Your sense of accomplishment can lead to a sense of aliveness. Allow *life* into your life. Experience a sense of community. When you feel that what is going on is overwhelming, complex, and complicated, notice the feeling and move on.

9.4.1 NORMALIZING THE PAY-OFF

If expectations get set, perhaps through old habit patterns, here is a way of dealing with them. An established expectation can be moved to an expectancy outcome pattern. The problem with expectations is that the outcome usually has a neutral or negative pay-off. How often does our life experience exceed our expectations? A way out of this problem is to normalize the pay-off so that all outcomes produce the same positive result. As follows:

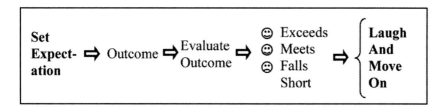

Reacting to Outcomes

Notice that in your movement toward your goals, the vision comes first, you apply actions toward a result, and the reality manifests over time. Be open to the process.

Remember to keep laughing at the outcomes! If the outcome is "Falls Short," moving on means we get to compare our results to our goal, note the differences, evaluate how our actions may have resulted in those differences, be grateful for the learning experience, plan new actions, and try again.

9.4.2 Laughing Off Stress

At one point several years ago, the stress I perceived in my life manifested as an ulcer. I stopped drinking coffee because I felt that I could handle coffee or stress, but not both, and I had more control at the time over drinking coffee. Eventually, as I was experimenting with ways to hold my life situation, I discovered that it was possible for me to take everything and everyone around me seriously but, at the same time, not take myself seriously at all. I was the joke in the middle of seriousness. With this viewpoint, my ulcer cleared up. I was able to get back to drinking coffee, which I love, and I was able to take on additional responsibilities because I was no longer particularly stressed about anything that was going on around me or within me.

If how you may do this is unclear to you, I invite you to go back and read section 4.2, "**Learning to Play**", on page 59.

9.5   THE VICE OF VICTIMHOOD

The next section is full of Useful Truths about how powerful we are that came out of a session when I was the client. I have since shared the information with my clients. We are all happy with the changes in our outlooks.

Presenting Issue:

Hello, Alan. It is nice that you can use your own techniques. We are all students here. Are there any emotional issues that you need to work on?

> "Sometimes situations get away from me and I just feel helpless. I do not like the feeling"

I know that being a victim is a learned behavior that does not have much value in life. I can notice when I feel helpless and make use of that feeling to motivate myself.

My father was a first generation American and a child of the Great Depression. He learned to deal with the feelings of victimhood by becoming immobilized. I saw, early on, how that approach did not work well for him and I vowed to take another approach. In the past, I have said to myself and others, "I don't do victim well!" I did not realize the hidden problem with that statement until now. It is now time for me to not do victim at all.

A new thought that comes up for me as I am writing this, "A victim is helplessly used by the world; a bodhisattva[50] is joyfully at service to the world. The difference is internal, so no one and nothing can get in the way."

Helplessness is the state where a person thinks that they have no choice. A person may or may not have any choice about their situation, but they always have choice about the way they feel. I know that over time my emotional state changes, there is always emotional movement. I seem to have no choice in that. I assert that I do have choice in the direction of my emotional movement. Some of the paths to travel are shown in the *Transforming Victimhood* box.

---

50 A bodhisattva is a being on the path to enlightenment. Enlightenment is freedom. Freedom is the goal of this book.

```
Helpless→Anger →Resolve→Action
Helpless→Depression →Apathy → Resolve → Action
Helpless → Acceptance → Resolve → Action
Helpless → Thoughtfulness →Consequences → Resolve → Action
```

Transforming Victimhood

I can still use more clarity on all the myriad guises of victimhood, so:

- My commitment is to give up what is not working.
- My commitment is to give up any victimhood about giving up victimhood.

Practice:

How does the *Transforming Victimhood* box make you feel? Is one of the patterns yours? Do you have a different road to action that I have not mentioned? The point is, when you feel helpless, do something (anything) about it. If you were lost in the woods and no one was looking for you, any direction could be the way out. When you are lost in your emotions, any movement allows the possibility of breaking out of your pattern.

9.6   MAKING I-DECLARATIONS

This section resulted from my taking my own advice. It deals with how a person's inner process spills out into the world.

Presenting Issue:

So Alan, how can you help yourself today?

> "When I am not with a client but just in everyday life, I try to share information in order to help another person. Their defenses go up and I do not have the impact I desire. It seems that I rarely am as helpful as I hope to be."

I am full of desires and way too close to myself to identify when I am acting out of altruism and when I have a hidden agenda. Whenever my world expands to include another person, the conversation between us become a co-creation[51] and within that creation, the border between where my influence ends and theirs begins can become complex. For example, as I speak, I may change my choice of words based on their changes in facial expression and they will usually wait for me to pause before they speak.

I know that I can only make a statement from my own viewpoint. Everyone else is in the same pickle. I can only hear a statement from my own viewpoint. Everyone else is in the same pickle.

Everything that happens to me may be considered as a metaphor[52] available for my personal growth. If I accept this as a Useful Truth, then, since hearing words is something that happens to me, I can conclude that all the statements I make or hear are actually statements about me in disguise! This sounds silly, but it may point the way to a very Useful Truth!

If I take the premise that all statements are also metaphors for personal growth to its logical conclusion, I may as well run the experiment of making a statement that is totally an expression of who I am. A declaration about me to me that clearly has nothing to do with anyone else. I will coin the term, "I-Declaration" for such a statement.

An I-Declaration is all about me. I do not need to share it with anyone else, although to distinguish it from normal self-talk and make it a declaration, I do have to speak it out loud or write it down. I may share it with a partner, but only out of compassion for them. My compassion may drive me to let my partner participate in and be cognizant of my inner space and my current challenges.

My I-Declaration is fundamentally different than the classic I-Statement[53] used in couple's therapy:

- Classic I-Statements are used as a non-judgmental communication tool to get *someone else to change* in order to improve a relationship while avoiding the assignment of blame.

- I-Declarations are used as a non-judgmental communication tool to define a level of *clarity to myself* while avoiding the assignment of blame.

---

51 This concept is developed by Dennis Rivers in *The Geometry of Dialogue: A Visual Way of Understanding Interpersonal Communication and Human Development*, available for free download at www.newconversations.net.

52 See Section 7.2.3 "Finding and Owning Misconceptions".

53 The classical formulation and use of I-Statements is provided in Appendix C.

9.6.1 FORMULATING I-DECLARATIONS

I notice that:

- An I-Declaration never requires action by another person.
- An I-Declaration never requires any change in the universe outside of me. In fact, it is a statement of current status and does not require change of any kind anywhere.

If I share my I-Declaration clearly, the person I share it with need not even acknowledge that they heard it! They have aided me as a sounding board. *Their inaction is a sign that I expressed the statement well.*

Now that I've shared, I can pay attention to what I said!

9.6.2 TESTING I-DECLARATIONS

Sometimes I have an issue with others around betrayal of trust.

An I-Declaration addressing this issue for me could be, "I am angry at myself for allowing the space around me to be used for betrayal. This self-anger supports my penchant to create myself as a victim."

That I-Declaration caused immediate movement in my world view, I experienced a sense of vertigo and I now have one less way that I get to victimize myself. My world keeps getting more bright and free.

Is there an I-Declaration that you can make that will release some negative emotion, concept, or memory that you have been holding on to? I invite you to run the experiment and see what happens. Maybe you can get dizzy too!

Maybe there is an "ah-ha" and a giggle waiting for you.

9.6.3 NOT I-DECLARATIONS

Attempting to make I-Declarations and listening to what actually comes out of your mouth can be lots of fun. Although they have a much different intent, I-Declarations are similar in construction to I-Statements. In practice, most I-Statements are actually "You-Statements" in disguise. I always enjoy hearing them. Here are a few examples:

- I feel that you are an idiot!

- I think that I would be better off without you!

- It is hard for me to make this relationship work on my own!

You get the idea. Since these are actually You-Statements, I have rewritten them to separate the "I" and the "you" components. The hidden I-Declarations in the above messages might have been:

- I frustrate myself when I attempt communication with someone who may not currently have the time, the interest, or the ability to hear me.

- I am not currently getting what I think I need out of our relationship. I had best get clarity and make a decision.

- I am feeling imbalanced in our interactions and the current split of responsibilities. I may have taken on more than I can handle at this time.

9.7 INNER CRITIC

Presenting Issue:

Good afternoon, Linda. What's up?

"You seem to have less trouble dealing with your inner critic than I do? Many times my inner critic sneaks in and sabotages my mood. Any ideas?"

The Dance of Ideas:

Here is a list of tips:

- When it shows up, I can take the opportunity to criticize my inner critic. "How lame are you? Is that the most negative comment you can make? You call yourself a critic! My mother could do better than you with no effort at all!"

- To the extent I carry my inner pattern outward, I have the opportunity to deal with my inner critic when I catch it critiquing others. If I can find gratitude toward the other, the critic shuts up.

- I can make the usually unsupportable assumption that my inner critic, no matter how screwed up, is trying to do what is best for me. From this position, I can love it and thank it for its help.

- I can use my inner critic as a coach or advisor. There is no point in reacting to it emotionally. I can just take corrective action as needed.

- I can put my inner critic on a stool in the corner and beam love toward it.

- I can say to my critic, "Thank you for sharing." I can accept that my inner critic is giving me another viewpoint that may add depth perception to the situation I find myself in.

- I can use my inner critic not to put myself down, but to find areas of improvement. The key is in how I formulate my inner questions. For example, "I am going to diet." cannot work for me personally because "diet" has "die" in it. It would be much better to ask, "How can I become lighter by creating new and satisfying meals?"

- When my inner critic shows up, I can welcome it and give it a useful task.

In summary I can:

- Dialogue with my inner critic.

- Find a positive in the message received. That is, take away any negative emotion and find the message for improvement.

- Consider my inner critic as a voice from the past. I can choose to deal with the present and let the past go.

Practice:

Use your observation skills to note when your inner critic shows up. Then apply one of the techniques above that seems appropriate.

I suggest that you experiment with the techniques that seem to you least likely to actually work, perhaps the technique that your critical facility thinks is ridiculous. You may be surprised at the outcome.

Chapter 10 Contents

Chapter 10 Figures

Chapter Ten
Sharing

10 SHARED FEELING

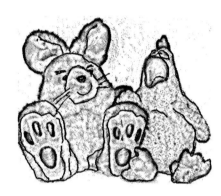

This chapter looks at the miscommunication of emotions that comes up when we interact with our partners and those to whom we are closest. It recognizes that our partners are worlds unto themselves.

Because emotions underlie so many of our interactions, it is useful to look at the emotional space we provide and receive from those around us.

I ask myself these questions regarding all my relationships.[54]

- How should I approach or stay away from my partners when they are looking moody and introspective?

- How well do I remember that the question I hear is not necessarily the question that is really being asked?

- What words and actions cause my partners to experience that they are loved by me? This is almost always different than the words and actions that cause me to feel loved by them.

- Do I hold my partners to a standard that I, myself, cannot meet?

- How serious should I be in my interactions with my playmates?

---

54 Relationships are usually thought of as between a person and a significant other. I am using relationship to mean between a person and **any** other. The moment I am interacting with anyone, parent, child, spouse, friend, or stranger, I am in a dance of relationship.

10.1   OUTER CRITIC

The real (outer) world is full of critics. Most folk find that it is easier to criticize a situation than to actually take corrective action. It is safer to critique than to attempt something that might fail. Having faced wounding criticism in our past can make us oversensitive in the present.

How may this rush to judgment affect our relationships with the people in our life?

Presenting Issue:

Hi, Linda. Do you have any responses to my suggestions on how to deal with your inner critic?

> "Yes, do you have some suggestions on dealing with *outer* critics? Sometimes I have seen compliments as a setup. Accepting the compliment leaves me vulnerable."

There is a technique in giving criticism that starts with a compliment. It is a one-two punch. For example, "I think that you are really smart. So why do you to do such dumb things!" Some possible responses are:

- I can accept a compliment and say, "Thank you." I can acknowledge the person complimenting me and deal with my feelings of vulnerability internally.

- Each statement made to me can be dealt with individually. "Thank you, I am glad that you consider me bright. I constantly attempt to think about my actions and make good choices. Please tell me how your perspective differs from mine." (Internally: If you cannot give me useful information, bugger off! You are not in a position to judge the wisdom of my actions!)

I remember from years ago, the concepts of warm-fuzzies and cold-pricklies.[55] The key is how you feel after receiving one. Sometimes a warm-fuzzy would be a cold-prickly in disguise. "You are really attractive for a fat lady!"

---

55   Defined as part of Transactional Analysis, as represented in the book *I'm OK, You're OK* by Thomas Anthony Harris.

I believe that compassion is the key in dealing with outer critics. If they are so critical of me, how critical are they of themselves? They may have to carry around an inner critic that is much more voracious than mine. I only have to interact for a time with them, while they are stuck with themselves 24/7. With this realization, my response to their criticism does not have to be anger or return criticism, but sympathy. From my sympathetic state, I can look to the content of their criticism and find the value for myself of being seen through the eyes of another.

Practice:

If you interact with other people for any length of time, ample chances will come up for you to practice sympathy, compassion, and forgiveness. Welcome to the human condition.

The exercise here is to wait for someone to criticize you. When this happens, assume that they mean well, leave your inner critic out of the loop as much as possible, thoughtfully evaluate what you have heard, and say, "Thank you."

If alarm bells go off for you and you cannot entertain for a second that they meant well, look at them with sympathy, and see if you can determine how often they criticize themselves in like manner. I notice that usually the sympathy is interpreted as interest or puzzled evaluation. This interpretation may be valid, because you may actually be both interested and puzzled. Your critic takes your look as a sign that you are honoring them by evaluating their input, which is, in fact, the case. They are ready to receive your response, which is, "Thank you."

10.2   PERSONAL STYLES AND WARNING SIGNALS

This section deals with our individual ways of organizing our minds and how we can make use of understanding our differences to aid in our communications with others.

Presenting Issue:

Good morning, Linda. What is your issue du jour?

> "Since we started working together, I have made tremendous progress in being a balanced, integrated, self-aware being. My balance[56] in my relationship with my partner and other people in the world, not so much."

I would like to provide some information on the way human minds work that may be of use to you. Next session we can work on learning your pattern and your partner's pattern and designing better ways for you to communicate with each other.

The Dance of Ideas:

Neuro-linguistic Programming™ (NLP) is the study of how the mind stores and processes information. There are three main ways, or modalities, that humans store sensory experience:

- visual (in our mind's eye)
- auditory (in our mind's ear)
- kinesthetic (in our body or our body image)

Visual information is easy to relate to as a picture. I might say, "Picture a cherry tree in first spring blossom. The wind blows the petals free and they drop toward the ground below." You call up or create a vision to match my words.

Or I might say something auditory, for instance, "Do you remember the words to God Bless America?" This brings up a voice in your head speaking or singing.

Or I might tie into something we store in our body image, "Imagine what it felt like to swing at a baseball." Or, "Are you hungry now?" What part of you did you access to obtain that information?

Our inner life is made up of the interplay of these different ways of relating to the world. The different representational systems are uniquely useful in different pursuits. As we grow up we each discover our own natural

---

56 This fuller level of integration proceeds as a natural consequence of our process of opening. Refer to the *Moving "Ouch-ward" and Growing* Box back on page 100.

pattern and this pattern supports our individual skill sets and allows us to become who we are as adults.

Habits are replays of procedural memories. Good spellers sound out the word that they are trying to spell (auditory), then see the word written on the blackboard (or whiteboard) in their head (visual)[57], then allow their hand to make the motions or their fingers to hit the appropriate keys in the proper order (kinesthetic). This pattern is obvious and similar for many people. The path to emotions and how we deal with them when relating to ourselves and others is much more complex and is different for different people.

There is a freeing Useful Truth here. Since most of our internal information processing is based on laid down habit patterns, recognizing our unique pattern in a given situation allows us to identify these habits and insert interventions that modify our process in useful directions. This technique will be demonstrated a few sections from now, after we expand our knowledge of modalities.

Practice:

Do you have a preferred style when solving a problem? Do you like to visualize a solution, state possible different outcomes with your inner voice, feel your way to a solution, or perhaps follow a pattern that mixes several of the above approaches in a pattern? Your pattern is unique to you and those around you will, most likely, have different patterns. Knowledge of a person's pattern is useful when trying to communicate with them.

Early in this book ("Finding Balance" practice on page 56) we introduced an exercise to help you find an early warning signal that could show up before any imbalance in your life would manifest as pain. What modality or pattern of modalities is associated with your signal?

---

57 English spelling has only a passing relationship to how words sound.

10.3 INTER-PERSONAL CONTROL ISSUES

Under continued stress and over time our personal boundaries can be worn down. Our loved ones can be inadvertently drawn into our suffering. Sometimes, actions that start out as attempts to help can become attempts to protect and control. Awareness and compassion can be the key to transformation of these incidents.

Presenting Issue:

Hi, Linda. Shall we continue discussing your issues with your partner?

> "Sometimes I feel like my partner is trying to control my every move. I feel sometimes that I have so little space of my own that I can hardly breathe."

The Dance of Ideas:

Linda, I invite you to use your finger-drop to go into trance and report your honest evaluation of the feelings underlying interactions with your partner.

> "The trauma of my accident and its repercussions had the effect of shaking my world and my partner's world. We had to adjust to a new reality. We had to face the reality that we might have lost each other forever.
>
> "Now there is an element of fear underlying our relationship that was not there before. I know that one of my responses to fear is to try to micromanage my relationships. I try to keep track of every part of my emotional environment. I want my partner to be predictable so that I stay in my comfort zone.

When I consider any political or social group that is fear-based, I notice that it members create rules to control behavior. Freedom is about determining our own behavior. Adult freedom means that we determine our own behavior in such a way that we are aware of the consequences of our actions for ourselves and others.

> "Now that my partner is called upon to be one of my caregivers, I think that I need him more than he needs me. My

fragility and my neediness frighten me. I know that almost losing me has frightened him.

"I know deep down that both he and I are trying to move away from our fear and back to a place where we feel safe and comfortable.

"I know that trying to control my partner does not work but I keep trying to do it.

"If I trust in the process that is us, rather than the process that is me, there is room for two viewpoints and both caregiver and care receiver are in a dance of love. Balance is a dynamic reality between us and neither of us has to control the other."

This space is worth cultivating.

Practice:

The idea that fear leads to an attempt to control is a Useful Truth.

These exercises cannot be simulated. Note the ideas and apply them when the chance arises.

1. When you find yourself trying to control[58] someone, ask yourself the question, "What am I afraid of?" and address the answer you get without attempting in any way to manipulate the other person.

2. When you find others trying to control[59] you, ask yourself the question, "What are they afraid of?", and address the answer you get as best you can without either allowing them to manipulate or reacting against their attempted manipulation.

---

58 In this case, control means trying to manipulate another person through threat, real or implied, through assertion of greater knowledge or status, real or implied, or through emotional blackmail. "If you loved me you would give me that last piece of pizza."

59 The clue that leads you to think someone is trying to control you is that you feel constricted in your body image. It is almost like they are trying to create a cage around you so you can only do what they want.

10.3.1 DESTRUCTIVE TESTING

Another take on the neediness issue runs like this: "He cannot really love me when I am this needy. I know that I do not love me this way. I find myself testing our relationship to prove that he will always be there for me."

This reminds me of two things. Frank Herbert states, in *Dune*, the first of his *Dune* series of science fiction books, "The proof that you have power over a thing is the demonstration of your ability to destroy that thing." In this case, the author was referring to the ecology of the desert planet that produced "Spice," a longevity drug. This destructive approach to life is ill-advised. It has no place in a healthy relationship.

The health of a relationship is not necessarily related to the physical health of the participants in that relationship. It is always related to the mental health of the participants.

This book has made no attempt to directly deal with anyone's physical health. That is what the medical profession is for. This book does provide information that allows for a freer, more vibrant, mental health and outlook.

Over the years, I have noticed that whenever I managed to make an improvement in my mental health (attitude), there was an immediate spill-over which seemed to increase the vibrancy and depth of all my relationships. Sometimes our improving mental health leads us in a direction we do not expect or maybe even realize that we want.

10.4   ANGER AS A CONFLICT OF STYLES

In this session, we continue to move our position in our dance with others. We move from fear to attempted control, to frustration, and ultimately to anger.

Presenting Issue:

Hi, Linda. How are your interactions with your partner, Jim, and the other people in your life improving or falling apart?

"I find myself getting angry and frustrated with the people around me. I ask myself, 'Why can't they be more like me?'"

The Dance of Ideas:

I would like to share some Useful Truths with you around the emotion of anger.

Some people do not feel safe expressing anger in the moment, while some do. Whenever it is expressed, non-destructively expressing anger is usually better than destructively holding it in.

When asked why he was not angry with the Chinese government for invading his country, the Dalai Lama responded, "I know of no Chinese person who would be hurt by my anger, but I know that I would be hurt!"

I find that a useful way to non-destructively express my anger is to use my anger to drive myself toward positive action. Anger then evaporates in service.

When I get angry, I can choose to assert the Useful Truth, "We are rarely angry at what we think we are." I then take the time to look underneath the anger. What I discover is usually a surprise and is always useful. I find my buttons and get to review their applicability in the current circumstances. Stated another way, anger at myself or someone else is a key to recognizing that a miscommunication is occurring.

I notice that there are at least two types of anger:

- **Clear Anger**—when we have clarity as to the cause within ourselves and are on-topic in dealing with the causes or expressing them to others.

- **Unclear Anger**—when we are in confusion. For example, I might bring in my parent's issues during a tirade about my current relationship issues. People tend to bring up past arguments with the person that they are currently angry with.

Practice:

Remember a time when you were verbally expressing anger. How clear was your expression? Is there a way that you could have made your expression more clear?

10.5 PERSONAL PATTERNS OF INTERVENTION

This section is an outgrowth of the realizations identified in the section relating to personal styles and warning signals (10.2 on page 177). Here identifying our interaction patterns within ourselves opens a window for changing our habits in life supporting ways. This means more opportunity to experience vibrant health.

Presenting Issue:

Hi, Alan, what issue would you like to work on today?

> "I want to gain mastery over what currently seems to be unconscious overeating."

The Dance of Ideas:

What do you have to say in trance?

> "I have the power to take control of my personal behaviors and change them almost immediately. The key is becoming conscious in time to make a choice."

This realization is worth expanding on. Most of our actions are governed by habit (a procedure we unconsciously follow), so all we need to do is insert a wake up call in the midst of the habit. The idea is to practice a common procedure and make a silly change. Then the change shocks us into becoming aware.

Since it disrupts any habit pattern, this technique can also be applied to help a person to stop smoking, to improve sports performance, or to avoid unnecessary fights with family or friends.

If I become aware of a way that I talk or a series of actions that always ends badly for me, I might as well stop that pattern early on. I have a story about this:

Once, after dealing with unexpected traffic, I arrived, hungry and tired, with my family at the hotel room where I proceeded to attempt to get my five-year-old daughter into a fresh outfit so we could dine. She was running and laughing and jumping on the bed. (I realize now that she was just unwinding her energy after being stuck in her car seat for several hours.)

I raised my voice as I tried to get control of the situation. My daughter looked at my rage-face and, wide-eyed, backed against the hotel room wall shaking.

My wife said, "I notice that you have scared our daughter. Was that your intent?"

"No, my intent was to get her attention. That did not require scaring her. In fact, I cannot think of any reason that I ever want to scare her."

In that moment, I was in touch with my driving emotion to control chaos and the realization that shouting adds to the chaos while calm humor and honesty has a chance of reducing it.

I learned how my parental pattern manifests and made an immediate change. From that time onward, when I feel that tight, get-in-control feeling in my lower stomach and the muscles tighten in my jaw, I breathe in to shout and I speak out with a calm measured request.

Nobody gets frightened and sometimes, to my surprise, my requests are honored.

That realization took the appropriate intervention of another person to wake me up. It turns out that I can apply the same intervention process to all the habits in my life that are not serving me well. I know that after about three bites of food I may have gotten enough to cover my energy needs. I also know that if I eat slowly I will enjoy the food more. I need to replace my tendency to gobble and gulp.

I analyzed how I eat food with a fork and added a silly self-intervention to help me break out of my eating habits. The new added intervention steps are shown in bold.

Eating intervention steps:

1. I cut a bite of my food with my knife or the side of my fork.
2. I feel the pressure of the plate against my utensil.
3. I pierce the food morsel with my fork and lift it to my mouth. *I am aware of the position of my hand around the fork.*
4. **Somewhere inside me there is a "one" count.**
5. I take my first bite.
6. I cut a bite of my food with my knife or the side of my fork.
7. I feel the pressure of the plate against my utensil.
8. I pierce the food morsel with my fork and lift it to my mouth. *I am aware of the position of my hand around the fork.*
9. **Somewhere inside me there is a "two" count.**
10. I take my second bite.
11. I cut a bite of my food with my knife or the side of my fork.
12. I feel the pressure of the plate against my utensil.
13. I pierce the food morsel with my fork and lift it to my mouth. *I am aware of the position of my hand around the fork.*
14. **As I move the morsel toward my mouth, somewhere inside me there is a "three" count. I lift up my forefinger and poke myself in the nose as I attempt to take my next bite! Ha!**
15. **With my silly poked nose action, I surprise myself into awareness. I consciously take my third bite and as I chew it, I evaluate how much I have eaten and how much more I may want.**

At this point I can choose to continue eating or to push the plate away and ask the waiter for a to-go box if I am at a restaurant. At home, I can put my plate in the refrigerator for later.

In a restaurant with friends, I stop eating and focus on the conversation. Usually no one seems to particularly notice my actions. If they comment on my reduced food intake, I respond that I am just not very hungry now.

I notice that at bite three, I sometimes stop eating, but usually continue. I notice that at bite six I usually stop eating, but sometimes continue. I notice that at bite nine I almost always stop, but sometimes chocolate cake can get the better of me.

I also notice that occasionally when I poke my nose I can surprise myself enough that I have to stifle a giggle.

Practice:

Try the above nose-poke intervention with a steak or a salad or some fruit. You can take very small pieces, so you can have many practice sessions before you are full. I recommend private practice, although I have noticed that people are rarely that observant, so I can usually get away with this in public. Have fun.

As an advanced exercise, try the intervention with a piece of cake. (I like this! I can eat as a part of my stop-eating practice! However, this excuse is short-lived!)

How would you apply this technique to eating a chicken drumstick?

How would you apply this technique to drinking a beverage?

It is generally easier to stop a habit pattern before it begins rather that disrupt one already in progress. Is there a habit that you have that you would like to eliminate or change? How early can you make the change? One client used the nose-poke approach to remind himself that he was a non-smoker each time he put a cigarette into his mouth. He would not light the cigarette, but, rather, take a deep breath and put the cigarette back into its pack. After a few weeks he stopped carrying around his pack of cigarettes and the habit of smoking was interrupted earlier in its pattern. After a few more weeks he no longer had any cigarettes in his life and the habit of cigarette smoking ceased to exist.

10.6　THE CENTER OF THE STORM

This session provides a Useful Truth and a visualization to help us stay centered.

Presenting Issue:

Hi, Linda. What's up?

> "I would like to have a visualization that I can use to help me weather the buffeting of life's storms that keep me from finding peace and rest."

I would also like such a useful image in this area. Let's kick around the idea and see what comes up.

The Dance of Ideas:

From my egocentric point of view, I am at the center of life's storms. Although I am in the world, I do not have to identify with the world. The word-image that comes up is, "I live in the calm and peaceful center of the storm while all around me swirl the thoughts, reactions, and plans that involve life's events." The events make life interesting, but I do not have to be emotionally drawn into them.

If we apply a hurricane metaphor we notice that:

- The more chaotic the hurricane, the larger the area of calm at the center.
- The winds move fastest just next to the calm. If a person were to step through the interface, they would feel twisted and jarred as part of their body is pushed by the wind and part is not.

This gives me an early warning system, a way of knowing when I am leaving the calm at my center. There is a sense of spinning or disorientation as I enter the maelstrom of my thoughts, a moment when part of me is still calm while part is now spinning. It is at that moment that I can choose to identify with and remain within my calm center, rather than be swept away by the drama of my life. I assert that it is possible to participate in life while remaining emotionally in the calm center.

Practice:

Exercise 1: I invite you to experiment with the visualization pictured in the *Staying in Our Calm Center* box. The little spinning arrows represent our disorientation as we move out of our center. The large rotating arrows represent the high wind near the center and the softer wind farther away. Do you notice that events far away have less influence on your equanimity than events in your neighborhood?

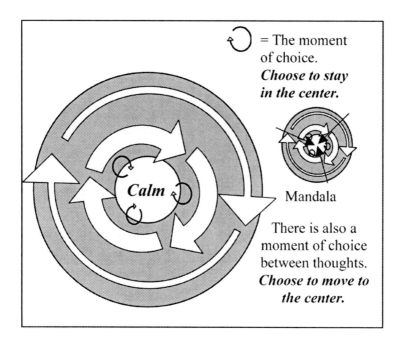

= The moment of choice. *Choose to stay in the center.*

Mandala

There is also a moment of choice between thoughts. *Choose to move to the center.*

Calm

Staying in Our Calm Center

If a person could stroll along within the center of a hurricane, he or she could view the maelstrom without being part of it. Similarly, we can view the events of our life drama without being caught up in them. The trick is to learn to recognize the moment of choice and then observe our drama without panicking and without identifying with it. This choice is represented by the arrows pointing the way back to the center of the mandala.[60]

---

60 Mandala is Sanskrit for circle, connection or community.

Exercise 2: Are you the participant of the events of your life or the observer of those events? You can run an interesting experiment to find out.

Please take a moment and respond to the following question as if I were facing you and asking it:

Who are you?

Notice the process that you go through in order to answer this question. Most folk go through a process similar to the following.

- Look back in memory at a series of sights-sounds-feelings from the past.
- Access a body image or sense of self.
- Bring it all together to formulate a short story, and
- Take a breath to speak.

So, who went through this process just now? Check it out again:

Who are you?

I would like to take this opportunity to say hello to the observer. That is who you really are! Sometimes, in the midst of action, you may be the participant as well, but you are always the observer.

The observer is independent of story. The observer is not tied to location. I assert that your observer is of the same essence (the essence of consciousness) as every other human's on the planet. From this perspective there is only one of us here. Heaven on earth comes from sharing and transcending our drama with caring others and being receptive to their sharing and transcending their dramas. Knowledge of other folk's drama expands us far beyond what we can cherish and experience with only one body.

Hell on earth comes from being tied too tightly to our own drama. That way lies fear of death, fear of loss, fear of change. I imagine that viewpoint prompted the Buddha to say, "All life is suffering."

In running the Center of the Storm visualization over time, I noticed an interesting transformation. There was an emotion living somehow inside/underneath/behind the Calm. The more times I chose to remain in the calm center, the more the calm transformed to joy.

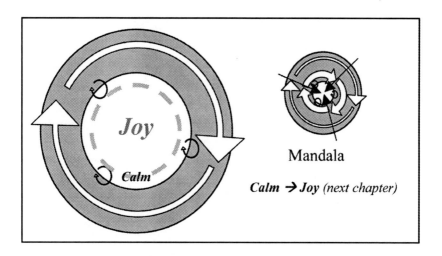

Inside the Calm

I now find myself inside the Mandala. There is more to come.

Chapter 11 Contents

Chapter 11 Figures

Chapter Eleven
Surprise

11 SURPRISES AT JOURNEY'S END

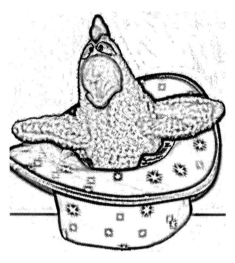

Welcome to the space of joy. It is time to manifest abundant, vibrant health.

This chapter reviews the path to this point, recalls the tools we now have available, and builds on them to achieve the freedom to live a balanced life.

In this chapter I summarize what Linda, my other clients, and I have learned in our time together. Sometimes the words in a section come from Linda's experience and sometimes they come from my experience or that of one of my other clients. We are dancing together as we talk about our insights. *I will use italics when I feel commentary is called for.* Read on, there are surprises still to come.

11.1   THE REALIZATION OF JOY

One day, the changes Linda had been making in her relationship to suffering took on a different flavor. Together we discovered the power of joy, something so simple and yet so profound that I needed to write this book so that I could bring it to you.

It was a joint realization and I do not know how it came into existence. I think that Linda asked if it was possible to change her way of living life, a daily practice that would not just transform her experience of pain, but would change her relationship to suffering in a way that would automatically move her toward balance without the need to even experience the pain part.

The direct application of joy, which is presented in Chapter 1, transforms those of us who are now using it. It resets our sense of self in a way that allows us to feel centered in comfort. We did not expand our comfort zone to include pain; life had already done that for us. We expanded our comfort zone to include joy and vibrant life entered us as a consequence.

11.2 THE GATEWAY TO ENLIGHTENMENT

The state of freedom that dwelling in joy brought us to caused us to think about enlightenment. One useful definition of enlightenment is freedom from identification with our story or, for that matter, any story; freedom from the tyranny of our own thoughts. Our thoughts are like objects on a table: we can order and re-order them; we can look at them; we can identify with them.

We are only one thought away from enlightenment and that is the thought that we are having right now. There is an opportunity in the small pause between thoughts to drop into an enlightened state, to drop into the silence between thoughts. Just as thoughts are objects on the table and silence is the table, we can choose to identify with our thoughts or the silence between them. We can be identified with the objects on the table or the table itself, the part of us that holds our thoughts.

I was honored to be present at the miracle when Linda, switching between outer-self and inner-self, had a conversation with her total being. I call the two voices Outer-voice and Inner-voice, other texts may refer to them as Observer and Participant.

11.2.1 HOW SUFFERING SERVES

Outer voice:

How did my suffering serve me?

Inner voice:

I have become who I am through suffering, through joy, through all life's events. Whenever possible, I choose joy. There is a spiritual that starts, "I've got that joy, joy, joy, joy down in my heart …"

What I am doing is allowing myself to be more self-aware. *Joy is freeing and freedom.*

Our positive experiences reward us and give us strength. Our negative experiences stretch us and teach us compassion. We need rewards, strength, stretching, and compassion to live balanced lives.

11.2.2 BALANCE OF FOCUS AND AWARENESS

Outer voice:

Sometimes I lose myself on the computer, or in any mental activity. Then, after a timeless time, I find myself feeling antsy and drained.

Inner voice:

The computer in front of me is like an extension of my central nervous system. As such, when I interact with it, my body awareness falls away and I get circulation/tension problems. My body likes to move. I am now at a place in my healing that my body has more energy than it had in the past. It needs to move to burn off some of that energy. I need to exercise every day. The antsy feeling is a message to exercise. Go for a walk. I have been striving for balance and I have to keep moving to be in balance.

11.2.3 TRUST

Outer voice:

I went through a trauma that took me to the point of death. And then I survived! The lesson I came away with is that I am afraid to trust life. How do I relearn trust?

Inner voice:

I started out trusting life, and I was right to do so. I am still here.

It is good to know that I can do hard stuff.

I do not want to repeat my trauma, even though I, on some level, do not know how to keep from doing that.

I can carry my lessons forward with joy to new beginnings.

I can use the experience as a reason to stop doing things that are bad for me.

11.2.4 ISOLATION

Outer voice:

In the midst of my lengthy hospital stay, I had a vision of a chain link fence with me on one side and the people I love on the other side. I tried to talk to them but they could not hear. I could not reach to them. I could not touch them.

Inner voice:

I am past that point now. Now I can take the time to *internally* express gratitude for the people in my life. As the occasion permits, I can take the time to *externally* express my gratitude.

11.2.5 ACHIEVING COMPLETIONS

Outer voice:

Balance is taking me toward completion. What do I need to say to the people in my life?

Inner voice:

I need to tell them I love them and have them get that. When that happens, I am complete. Tomorrow, I may want to do that again, but if there is no tomorrow it is OK. Completion is about loving them enough to let them go on their own paths.

Outer voice:

This feels like I turned a corner and I am heading off in a new and good direction for myself.

Nobody said it would be easy. But notice: If we love a person enough to let them go, there is no clinginess left in the relationship. Then we are free to really experience our love for them because it is not tainted with fear. Our love is fully in the moment.

11.2.6 INDIVIDUAL ENLIGHTENMENT

Outer voice:

Can I summarize all that I have learned to this moment regarding individual enlightenment, regarding pain, death and separation?

Inner voice:

Everyone else is a metaphor for my own internal work.

I am grateful that I have loved people so much that their leaving hurts, leaves such a hole in my life.

Extend it "I love myself enough to let me go, to drop my own act. I am not my act." This is the road to peace.

Practice:

Can you let go of your act without judgment? I invite you to run the experiment.

Here are some suggestions for practice during the weeks to follow. The basic plan is to focus on our joy and to physically exercise when we get the chance.

Attempt to tune in sooner, at the very beginning of the pain.

Give yourself a little slack; remember that a habit is hard to break. Even if you do not want it, it becomes part of who you are.

In his poem "The Prisoner of Chillon" Lord Byron said, "My very chains and I grew friends …" It is time for some new friends.

11.3   MOVING OUTWARD TO OTHERS

Linda continued to share her realizations with me. Now she was wide awake and her eyes were wide with shock and pleasure.

"In the middle of my Joy exercise I notice that the Joy takes flight!

"There has been a shift from: 'Pain is starting and I must take something' to 'Pain is starting and I will wait and see what happens.' I notice that two out of three times, pain goes away on its own without medication!

"I am strong enough now to consider being a support to the other people in my life who have been supporting me. As I celebrate this moment, I consider and accept this useful viewpoint: I stand in humble awe of the part of God that I am."

Yes, Linda, now that you have a solid experience of your calm center, you can allow this calm to expand to include another person.

This is pictured in the *Expanding Your Calm Center* box. I have discovered that I can accept another person from my center of calm. In fact, the measure of how well I am centered during an interaction is how tired I feel after the interaction. If I stay out of judgments and parenting there is nothing emotional to feel tired about. The interaction does not take much mental energy and little energy needs to be replenished. In fact, it is possible to feel energized and enlivened by the experience of sharing.

During any interaction your calm center can expand to include the other person and then your version of their drama evaporates. In the space of magic, their version of the drama also evaporates! This happens not because of anything you do as much as because of your inner peace communicating and spreading itself.

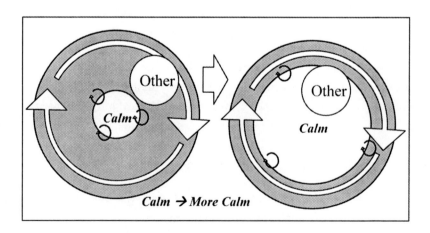

Expanding Your Calm Center

Practice:

This exercise takes another person and a disagreement or at least a feeling of discord. I do not recommend that you intentionally create such a situation. Just review the exercise so that when the situation arises, you are prepared to behave in a new and potentially rewarding way.

Recognizing boundaries is a sign of good mental health. In this exercise we honor other people's boundaries while emotionally inviting them to experience joy with us. Refer to the *Expanding Your Calm Center* box for a visualization of the process. Read over the steps a few times so that you will be ready to run through them when you have the occasion and this book is not handy.

1. The key to starting this exercise is recognizing the feeling of spinning disorientation that occurs when you reach the border of your calm center ("Center of the Storm" practice on page 189.)

2. For a moment ignore the outside world and move to establish yourself within your calm center.

3. From this calm center look at your partner in this dance of discord. With no physical movement, reach out and cherish them.

4. With no judgments or words or deeds welcome them to join you in calm.

5. While maintaining your sense of calm, allow your sense of identity to expand so that you and your partner are co-creators of a dance. Identify with the dance rather than either individual. This allows a space of balance. A dance works when both partners are in balance. Graceful movement happens when both are in synch.

6. Given the chance, your partner will most likely follow your lead and join you in calm.

7. If your calm spreads, notice it in your partner's body relaxing. Do not claim anything or say anything that might disrupt the shared moment. Just notice it and be grateful.

8. If your calm does not spread this time, be grateful that at least you can experience it. Hold your space and be prepared to run the experiment again at the next opportunity.

9. From your position of gratitude, say whatever comes up to say or implement whatever actions come up to do in order to express and validate the calm that is you.

11.3.1 HELPING SUFFERERS

In my hypnotherapy practice, people come to me and present an issue. My intention is to be of service in a way that brings them relief. I maintain my calm center as I attempt to take on a person's burden of pain and suffering.

- I hold the burden for a time.

- I notice its weight while remaining separate from its impact.

The person has the space to experience life without the burden. They may later take it back up or not. The burden may not have changed but the person has.

11.4   PAIN MANAGEMENT SUMMARY

Pain is a boundary. We can choose to go beyond it.

Pain is sensory experience interpreted with a fear-induced sense of separation. Since our sense of identity is different than the pain, we can perceive the source of pain as being outside of us, even though it is within our body.

What we experience is in the map of our body that exists within our head. We have the freedom to change our relationship to that map.

Recall (Chapter 5) that there are four direct ways of handling pain:

- Ignore it.

- Focus elsewhere.

- Honor and accept it.

- Tighten focus on it.

Honoring the pain allows us to use it as a tool for our self-growth. We can use self-hypnotic trance work in conjunction with any of these approaches.

Chronic pain is different than occasional pain. The chronic pain experience is: Chronic Pain → tired → cranky → more pain, while the occasional pain experience is: Pain → action → no pain, where the action may be to do something, like pull a splinter out, or to take something, like an aspirin.

We can also experience that Pain → Tension. Where does an individual hold their tension? *I assert that it is possible for a person to hold their tension outside of their body.* Then they can choose to let the tension go or to hold it in new and interesting ways. To accomplish this they may have to look at the underlying beliefs that keep them holding on to their tension.

From the state of expectancy, a person's emotional reaction to events outside of their control is to be thrilled! *I am swept off my feet. I live in a new and different, wondrous place where, once again, anything is possible. I am taken out of my comfort zone, out of the place where I thought I knew what was going on.*

11.4.1 THE PAIN BALL

There is a great technique that is a result of the realization that I can hold my tension or any pain I am experiencing outside of my body. Since I experience the pain only in the map of my body that exists in my mind as part of my self-image, it is possible to:

- Interpose a pain-valve between my awareness and the experience. The pain comes from the same place but it is less strong. This is very useful and was described as a practice in section 5.2.

- Move the experience to another part of the map. A pain in one part of my body can be experienced in another part. Since it can be moved around, it is possible to move the pain off the map *entirely*! Achieving this may take some focused practice[61], but it is a useful,

---

61 Focused practice is something that our finger-drop technique can help us with.

powerful, and fun-to-use skill to possess. Since I discovered that I can hold my tension outside my body, I no longer suffer tension-related backaches, stiff necks, or headaches.

Here is the process that takes advantage of holding pain experience outside my body.

Suppose that I need to keep track of my pain. For instance, I am at the doctor's office and I am asked to rate my pain level from one to ten. I can do the following:

1. I create a pain ball as a holding area outside of my body. I make mine the size and shape of a blue bowling ball that floats weightless at waist height in front of me and to the right. I can keep track of it there.

2. If I have not already done so, I move my pain experience into the ball. My ball stays blue, but some clients have noticed that their ball changes color to red or orange when the pain is placed inside.

3. Now I can look within the ball and rate the pain level.

Additionally, now I can actively participate in the search for any physical reasons for the pain. I can actively participate in physical therapies to alleviate the physical causes of the pain symptoms. I do not have to be bothered by the pain, since it is not directly connected to me.

11.5   STAYING BALANCED AUTOMATICALLY

Linda and I find that we are now automatically performing a periodic Self-check-in. We find ourselves naturally taking actions that promote our good health. We find ourselves making food choices based not on what will feel good to eat, but on how we will feel later.

"I now act as if I am going to succeed, as if I am taking flight."

Practice:

Remember that you have an easy way to achieve a life-affirming trance state by use of your finger-drop. Think about what trance work you would like to do in order to move forward. What does moving forward mean to you in this context?

11.6   CHRONIC PAIN MANAGEMENT

A person experiencing a trauma assumes that this is a temporary state. We feel that we will somehow return to our previous state, but sometimes this is not the case.

When someone doesn't feel well for an extended period of time, they do not get to be the person they want to be. They are irritable, less flexible; they have less reserve, and less patience. Their relationships are affected as the pain wears on them day by day.

Chronic Pain ←→ Chronic Weariness

It is easy to get enmeshed in this loop. In the past, Linda became hypervigilant[62] because she so often felt fragile. She experienced that:

Hypervigilance ←→ Chronic Weariness

Easy things became hard things and she no longer felt that she was in charge. Hypervigilance took over and fed itself. Pain became an end in itself. That was the way it was! That is not the way it is or the way it has to be! Now she has the tools to maintain a state of vibrancy, immediacy, and high energy. *Tension is outside of my body, vitality is inside.*

Practice:

Remember the joy that comes just before the giggle. Let it fill you. Let it relax you. Let it wash away the fatigue. Giggle.

11.7   PAIN BALL AND MAELSTROM REVISITED

The calm at the center of life's storm can be viewed in three dimensions. We can combine the pain ball and the hurricane visualizations. Then we can view pain from our body through the pain ball and suffering from life as buffeting from the maelstrom outside our calm. The maelstrom does not touch us and we can moderate our internal experience by moving the pain ball, as necessary, as far from us as we desire. The calm at the center of the

---

62   Hypervigilance can be a symptom of codependency, which addressed briefly a few sections from now.

hurricane extends all the way to the stratosphere, no matter how far away we move our pain ball, it still floats in place, available to us, yet isolated from life's storm.

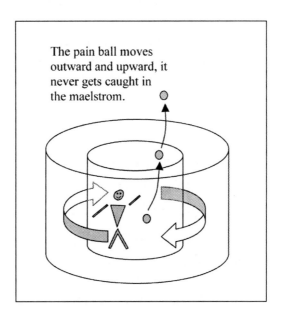

Above the Maelstrom

It is also possible to just drop the pain ball and walk away.

11.8 Death, Control, Fear, & Codependency

In this section I refer to the situation where one person allows another to control their feelings as codependency.[63] It is about boundaries. As social beings, our emotional worlds are impacted by and have impact on the worlds of others. A desire to please others is a normal part of existence. A need for interaction with others is a natural part of adult life.

---

63 Clinical codependency that leads to inappropriate forgiveness of abuse and attempts to control other adults or allow other adults to control us is outside the scope of this book. If you find yourself in such a situation, please seek professional help.

The border between healthy interaction and codependency is the boundary of suffering. When we are finding fulfillment and getting joy out of our interactions this is healthy. When we are finding pain, something has gone out of balance.

Individuals with chronic disabilities and their support team must constantly struggle against codependency. It is an easy trap to fall into. The way to avoid it is to periodically check how we feel about our situation.

One of the ways children are taught about appropriate behavior is with the statement, "If it feels wrong, it probably is." Co-dependent situations leave a bad taste in the mouth!

Neuro-Linguist Programming™ (NLP) provides the concepts of the behavioral model and behavioral meta-model:

- Our behavioral model consists of how we think we should behave.

- Our behavioral meta-model consists of how we think that everybody else (the mysterious and nebulous "they") thinks we should behave.

One cannot get milk at a hardware store, or love from a person unable to provide it. We can work on realizing this but there is always the hope that a person or situation will change.

Ah-ha: The last curse let out of Pandora's Box[64] was hope. This is the most subtle and most dangerous curse. It leads to continued co-dependency. Hope can be a blessing, in that it can provide a ray of sunshine in an otherwise bleak outlook. It can also be a curse, in that it can keep us way too long from taking action to rectify a suffering-filled situation.

My fears tell me that if I love a person, I open myself to the pain of separation when I am not with them. This may sometimes be the case, but if I can pay attention to happiness when it comes around and minimize paying attention to the pain and suffering when it comes around, I come out ahead. No one makes me pay attention to my drama! I get to choose.

---

64   In Greek mythology, Pandora was the first woman. She opened a container releasing all the evils of mankind, greed, vanity, etc., and leaving only hope inside. Hope was released later.

11.8.1 ENLIGHTENMENT 101: OWNERSHIP

I remember that I am the owner of everything inside myself. Everything that happens outside of me is just a (Useful Truth) metaphor that can be used for my inner growth. This means that only I-Declarations reflect the truth of me for me.

A Useful Truth for me is that my behavior is not predicated on or designed to cause any particular behavior in other adults. When I accept this as a way of being, it makes my victimization of myself and/or others impossible. Certainly, an evildoer could victimize me, but internally I am always free to choose alternative interpretations of my predicament that may provide me a creative way to gain control of a situation.

The statement, "I need you to give me a hug." is co-dependent. The statement, "I need a hug. Would you care to supply one?" is not.

Learning to experience life as an I-Declaration is an ongoing challenge. Enlightenment goes against my early training!

11.9 ENERGY BLOCKS

Linda and I realize that now virtually unlimited mental energy is almost always available to us. Energy seems to flow into us from the universe and we apply it to action. If this process is not happening to our satisfaction, it is useful to ask the question, "What is the block?" There is either a block between us and our energy or a block between us and our willingness to take action. We just need to focus on the area and ask the question, "What is the block?" then see what comes up. The reasons that come up are always useful.

Practice:

If you choose to practice this exercise, there are a few rules that help it be effective:

- Be willing to acknowledge and thank yourself for your inner honesty.
- Resist judging or criticizing yourself, remember that the child within you is a child that may have selfish needs that need to be addressed.
- Honor whatever comes up and decide how to address it.
- Remember that a decision to not act is also a valid decision.

11.9.1 FAITH

Going into trance, Linda asked, "How do I make a habit of continuing to celebrate the opportunities to experience compassion, abundance, grace, and joy in my life?" And the answer she received was, "It is there for the taking. It is not something that has to be dug out."

A trance is not always necessary. *I notice that when I am in touch with myself, asking the question brings an immediate result.*

We have experienced that life events, circumstances, interactions, aches and pains are objects on the table of our awareness. Joy is the table.

In Exodus 16:4-19, the Biblical manna and faith story, the Israelites are given exactly the amount of food they need each day. No more and no less. They cannot save for another day. They have to trust that a sufficient amount will always be provided. It is a test of faith.

We remember that all the people in our life are part of our team. They supply energy and at times we get swept up in their energy. This realization leads us to enlightenment 102.

11.9.2 ENLIGHTENMENT 102: COMPASSION

What I, and most adults, have done up to now is:

> When someone interacted with me and it did not go well, I would end up feeling bad about the interaction.
>
> I already know that blaming others is a waste of time. In my search for good feelings, I would then go inside myself to discover the problem.
>
> It would usually turn out that there was a miscommunication in my life metaphor. I would resolve the issue internally and I would feel OK.
>
> Then I could move on with my life.

Now:

> If my compassion so moves me, I can make an I-Declaration regarding the interaction and address it to the other person. This can be a test of my completeness. If I no longer have

an issue in this area, I will be able to communicate effectively with the other person. They will be able to hear me and choose to modify their behavior in the world or not.

The idea is that the other person does not have to change. In order to formulate a clear I-Declaration, I have already grown and changed enough to accommodate or at least to tolerate their behavior! They are presented with feedback that they may never have been effectively given before. If they so choose, they have the opportunity to change their behavior so that in the future they can communicate better with people like me.

I am not attached to the interaction and have no investment in the outcome. This level of communication does not come about often, but when it does, it is thrilling!

11.10 NEW BALANCE

We have had the experience that negative emotions and thoughts can be held in containers outside of our body.

Our emotions can transform if we give them a chance:

Fear → Curiosity

Pain → Anger → (turn Anger into Power)

Passion + Curiosity → Creativity "Messy is OK."

"I can get out of the container that is me. I do not have to have a specific shape. If this means that I am unknown that is OK."

Good! Be a mystery!

When life is good and we are feeling in balance, we can just stay with it. When any pain or suffering comes into our awareness, we can drop into the mystery.

We started on a quest to achieve balance. We can become so wide that we are solidly stable and cannot be anything but in balance.

Earlier on this journey we held the image of a tightrope walker balancing. That got us to now. Now we may be ready for a new image.

A possible new image is:

> I am supported by a riverbed that guides, protects, and sustains me as I flow. It contains me without limiting me or being a barrier. I can notice life's events and flow right on.
>
> I can be amorphous, containing nothing solid enough to receive a blow from the world. The "spears and arrows of outrageous fortune" pass through me and I am untouched.

11.11 EXPLOSION OF BEING

Linda has found a new way of being.

"I no longer experience limitations with passive impatience. My experience of them has moved through frustration to active anger and rage, for which I can find positive outlets.

"I now experience myself as an explosion full of light, energy, and enlightenment.

"I can:

> Let it be big
>> Let it go
>>> Let it rage
>>>> Let it move
>>>>> Let it explode!"

"As I reside in a space of bliss, I allow the explosion to happen."

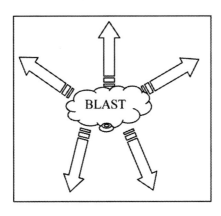

11.11.1 ENLIGHTENMENT 103: CHILD WITHIN

Any number of infant me's and child me's are inside me, alive and vibrant. We are one. Inside me now:

- I am the caregiver
- I am the care receiver

All else is illusion.

In this place pain has no space. It is just part of the oneness. What a relief!

11.11.2 THE PATH TO COMMUNITY

Linda noticed that passion and excitement, where it involves doing outer things that she is still not able to do herself, is still an edge of her comfort zone.

Before her accident, Linda was independent. Since then, she was dependent until we started working together.

Now she can move to a place where she is interdependent. She can move and give and receive easily.

Being in that space is not hard. The struggle to allow herself to be in that space can still be hard.

"This is another big corner. I have really been hungry for this space and I am thankful for it. I feel like this is my soul speaking.

"*Blast* → I have moved from Joy to Bliss."

The center and the moving out is everything. Energy is totally free in the *Blast* space.

11.12 CELEBRATIONS

Linda said. "I am part of a women's group that has met weekly for years. They reported to me, 'This is the first time that you have talked about your pain without it being a negative statement about you!' Pain and its accompanying limitations do not define me any more!"

"I am getting to the place where pain/fatigue is not the definer/limiter. It is just information!"

"Comfort/support/balance/maintenance has transformed and become strengthening/going forward."

"My life experience has moved beyond balance to freedom. It has moved beyond joy to contentment."

Yes! Our goal was always freedom, our path to get there led through balance. Our tool to maintain balance is the joy that comes just before the giggle. The end result is contentment, a happy resting place. The emotion associated with the starting place that is shown for the baby pictured in the diagram in Chapter 1.

"The image of me as a flowing river (earlier in this chapter) is compelling. I can trust my inner feelings and move forward untroubled by the past. Events and emotions are just ripples in the stream."

As Scarlet O'Hara said in *Gone with the Wind*, "… tomorrow is another day."

This thought set Linda up for another explosion:

Blast →!! Again, she moved from Joy to Bliss.

11.13 EPIPHANIES

It is helpful in looking at the world and our place in it to remember that at the level of the non-conscious mind, things are organized in a different way:

- In the external world or its map, objects are related to other objects by space/time position or attribute.

- In the internal world, concepts are organized by emotional context.

We mused on the children in our life and recalled from *The Prophet*, by Kahil Gibran, "Your children are not your children, but are beings of light entrusted to your care for a time." This thought brought us to enlightenment 104.

11.13.1   ENLIGHTENMENT 104: NON-ATTAINMENT

I am not my own to keep. I am what was entrusted by the divine to my care. *I am mine to care for, cherish, and enjoy!*

In summary, I have moved from dealing with the chronic pain of a physical/medical situation to confronting the pain of being human. The pain of being human will be with me as long as I choose to remain human.

11.13.2   ENLIGHTENMENT 201: I AM THE WORLD

The enlightenment class numbers jump to 201 because this epiphany moves us out of identification with our body and into identification with all of humanity!

There is only one of me here. I can choose to identify myself as all-of-the-world with my center not necessarily inside my body and listen to what I am telling myself.

What am I asking for? What is being asked of me? How may I be of service to the divine in this moment?

This question sometimes receives the answer, "Keep doing what you are already doing." And a mundane everyday activity turns into holy action. Suddenly, I dwell in grace and I am reminded to laugh at my pretension.

- If I take myself seriously, life becomes work and my self-importance becomes a burden to carry. I hear my inner voice to the exclusion of the myriad outer voices and fall from grace.

- If I hold myself lightly and full of giggles, life becomes play and I have no importance, only humility in the face of the divine seen in both the world of nature and the world of man. My feelings about the messages I receive from the world and my feelings about the messages I receive from myself mesh and I live in grace.

11.13.3   ENLIGHTENMENT 202: I AM

!

Surprise

Chapter 12 Contents

Chapter 12 Figures

Chapter Twelve
Balance

12 MAINTAINING BALANCE

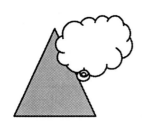 As discussed in the last chapters, if we are at our calm center, our vision of balance may no longer look like trying to stand up straight. We may see ourselves as a pyramid with a wide solid base or as a cloud floating in the sky where balance has no meaning. From this vision of stability how do we move toward our goals?

The river analogy presented in the last chapter frees us from constantly driving ourselves toward our goals. We can just be the flow and know that eventually we will reach our destination. This visualization allows a dynamic model of rest. Movement toward our goals never has to stop. Our goal setting and our intention has created the bed of our river of being. We move along and enjoy the scenery while our intention adjusts the channel that exists just beyond the next bend. We do not have to worry about or even to see what is coming. We will get there in due time.

12.1 THE TARGET AND THE PATH

We are always involved in the dynamic creation of our future. This section provides an effective creation process. A few helpful affirmations are provided below:

- With each breath I have the opportunity to continue learning new ways of being.

- I am the only one who creates my experience of reality.

- I can find a feeling placed around what I want and the feeling will lead me to the actualization.

- Just seeing a few hundred feet ahead to the next bend is sufficient to get me to my destination.

The process can be pictured as shown in the *Bliss Creation Circle* box.

Manifesting success in the world can be quite easy, in spite of many experiences that contradict this. The space for success is created by the process, then success manifests. This is hard to accept at face value, but it is worth running the experiment and testing the process.

The process proceeds when we let our bliss drive our learning, which drives our creativity, which drives our dreams and goals, which drives creation, which is the manifestation of our bliss.

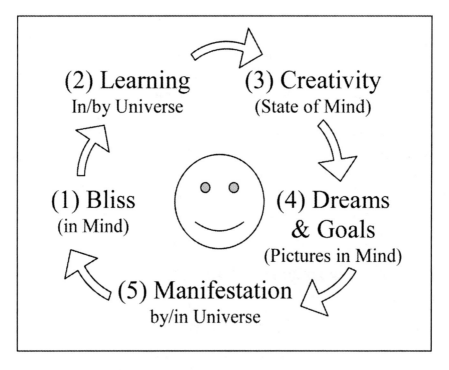

Bliss Creation Circle

In the *Bliss Creation Circle* box, we start at (1) and allow the rest to happen. The process is not a circle, but rather a spiral upward. Each time around, bliss is reinforced.

Another way to view this process is that most people think, based on early childhood training in this society, that they must **do** something so that they can **have** something, and then they will **be** something. The box shows that this understanding is flawed compared to the way that the universe of human society actually works.

A more effective process is first, **being** in a state of bliss as shown at location (1); this leads to **having** the experience of learning, creating, and identifying dreams and goals (2, 3, 4), and ultimately **doing** or manifesting the actions (5) that appear from the outside to lead us to our bliss. From the inside, the manifestation is actually doing what comes naturally at that point of the process.

12.2 GRATITUDE

Opportunities to understand and experience gratitude keep showing up in my life. A French proverb states, "Gratitude is the heart's memory." Expressing gratitude is remembrance of our interconnectedness with others, a confession of our humanity, and a way of recognizing that we do not walk alone.[65]

I am so happy and grateful now:

- That I have the knowledge and freedom to create each day new and alive.

- That I have sufficient health and resources to start any enterprise and the universe will joyfully augment and support my actions.

- That I have people to care about.

- That my sense of humor has survived intact since childhood.

- That each moment my giggle grows to include more people.

---

65 From the Rev. Dr. Louise-Diana. I subscribe to her on-line *Inner-Fitness* newsletter and received this around Thanksgiving, 2006. Her web site is www.inner-fitness.com.

- That the people around me consistently model for me better and clearer ways of being.

- That the world abounds with my friends.

- That I have the chance to clean up my interactions.

- That I get to share a vision of freedom with you!

12.3 BALANCE IN YOUR BODY

This book has presented concepts that, for the most part, are thought experiments designed to help a person take charge of their emotional experience of life. This section presents a direct movement exercise that allows a person to use their body image directly for physical healing work.[66] It allows the possibility of naturally finding new ways to balance the physical body; just as previous chapters allow the possibility of new ways of holding and balancing relationship with life.

Thinking about moving a muscle may produce micro movements in that muscle which integrate the mind and body in more subtle ways than are produced by the gross muscle movements we use to get around. This technique builds on that possibility. The practice provided as an example helps relieve the symptoms of a stiff neck. Generally one side is stiffer than the other.

---

66 My exercise is based on the Feldenkrais technique or method, bodywork developed in Israel by Russian-born Israeli educator Moshe Feldenkrais, D.Sc. (1904-1984). His method establishes new connections (or reinforces old working connections) between the brain and body through movement re-education.

Feldenkrais proposed that nearly our entire spectrum of movement is learned during our first few years of life, but that these movements represent a mere 5 percent of all the movement possibilities available to us. Habituated responses to problem areas in our lives may be ingrained in our movement patterns. By retraining the central nervous system through skeletal system movements similar to those in the exercise presented, old patterns may eliminated and replaced with new skills that improve the physical, mental, and emotional functioning of the body. In this way, unconscious movement is brought into conscious awareness where it may be used as a tool for healing.

Practice:

Stiff neck reduction exercise:

1. Stand straight with arms hanging freely, feet spread and in line with shoulders, face centered to the front.

2. Picture what it would be like to slowly rotate your head and body to the right and back to center. How far would your head go? How far would your shoulders go? How far would your hips go? What would the sensations in your head, neck, shoulders, upper back, lower back, buttocks, upper legs, lower legs be? How would your hands and arms swing?

3. Run the experiment by actually rotating to the point of pain or a natural stop and coming back to center. Compare your picture and your reality and note any discrepancies.

4. Adjust your picture and run through step 2 and step 3 again.

5. Repeat steps 2 though 4 a third time to see how close you are. Notice that the degree of swing in the third pass has most likely increased somewhat from the first pass.

6. Repeat steps 2 though 5 for a rotation to the left and back to center. Notice that the rotation toward one direction is more flexible than the other.

7. Focus on the more flexible, less painful side. Facing front, picture what the feeling of slightly raising (micro movement of 1/4 to 1/8 inch) that shoulder would be in your body image.

8. Test the non-stiff side against your image.

9. Run the process (steps 7 and 8) a few more times to get it solid in your mind.

10. Pause for several seconds to allow your right side feelings to move to your left side and vice versa.

11. Picture what micro movements in your formerly stiff side would feel like.

12. Your exercise is done. Do not bother to test the stiff side image!

13. Go about your day. Notice that you have less restriction and freer movement overall.

As you practice this technique, allow yourself to feel excitement with the process of creation and change that happens within your body.

Although I cannot speak from my own experience in this area, I have been told by people who have had direct experience that the technique of periodically picturing, as fully as possible, the movement of a limb while that limb is immobilized in a cast, results in a retention of muscle tone and a radically shortened recovery time once the cast is removed.

12.4 ON AGELESSNESS AND AUTHENTICITY

There is a rhythm to authenticity. It includes the heart. How easy it is for me to hide from myself. The juice is in my commitment to finding and dealing with the dark and the light of my life. If I can create a space where I do things simply for my inner joy, then I can be congruent in my life. There is an extra benefit if others who I care about also get joy.

As I live from that space and follow my muse, I become ageless. I am free to follow any path and all paths that come my way. I am free to have any story, no story, or all stories. I am free.

I choose to live every moment just before the giggle.

I invite you to join me.

Afterword
Finding Grace

One Useful Truth goes, "When the student is ready, the teacher shows up."

In the text that follows I share the mystery of my personal experiences involving a spiritual master by the name of Swami (Baba) Muktananda. All events are reported as accurately as I can remember them. In the years after I met him an organization called The Siddha Yoga Foundation grew up around Baba. It continues to spread his teachings and preserve his spiritual lineage.

I am not a joiner and have no connection to the organization. I follow my own path. I am willing to listen to others and I am willing to experiment with any spiritual practices that make sense to me. I do not believe in following any person or adopting any practice blindly.

Throughout this book I provided explanations and suggested harmless (no-downside) experiments. I neither advocate nor refute any of the practices suggested by Baba, his disciples, or their organization. I am just sharing some of my experiences around the man himself.

At the Feet of the Guru

I met Swami Baba Muktananda at a lecture presented at the Whole Earth Festival at the University of California Davis campus in 1973[67].

I learned of the event from a friend of mine who followed the spirituality scene and suggested we meet him. We sat on a blanket on the floor of a

---

67 The **Whole Earth Festival** is a three-day music and education festival in the spring. It usually takes place during Mother's Day Weekend on UC Davis' main quadrangle. Every year, thousands of environmentally conscious, politically active and/or music-loving people make the pilgrimage to Davis for this event, for which the UCD quad is filled with hundreds of craft booths, music acts, education booths, and food booths.

gymnasium with a stage at one side: my friend, my young son Raymond, and myself.

Baba turned out to be a small bearded man who wore a saffron robe and spoke in Hindi which was translated by a shaven-headed monk who was always at his side.

He sat before the group answering questions and telling stories. He laughed a lot and so did the audience. I found myself laughing until tears poured out of my eyes. I knew intellectually that I was just viewing a strangely dressed little man, but somehow he was a bright blue point of light that was almost too bright to look at. Have you ever been in a situation where you have the thought, "Something wonderful is happening here that I do not understand?"

Baba and Divine Nature

On an early visit to Baba's new ashram[68] in Oakland I got lost and found myself in a corridor off the main meditation hall. In front of me approached Baba. As a newbie, I did not know how to behave. Should I bow? Should I step aside? I stood there dumbly. Baba, his translator, and I were alone together in the silent passageway.

Baba grabbed my upper arm and spoke into my ear. His ever-present translator, Dr. Jan, grinned and spoke into my other ear. Although I stand a head taller than Baba, I felt like I was a seven-year-old held up on tip-toe by a parent and powerless to move in an iron strong grip.

Baba whispered something in Hindi into my left ear.

Dr. Jan said into my right ear, "He said to tell you he is God!"

Baba whispered some more.

Dr. Jan, "He said that he does not expect you to take his word for it. He expects you to test his presence in your life."

Baba grinned and whispered some more.

Dr. Jan, "If and when you are sure he is God, come back and visit him. He says he has a message for you!"

---

68 An ashram is the dwelling place of a Guru or teacher; a monastic retreat site where seekers engage in spiritual practices and study the sacred teachings of yoga.

Baba winked, released me, turned and walked away.

Well, I consider myself an engineer. For years I tested in every way that I could imagine. Some of these Baba stories come from those tests. Finally I was convinced. I asked Baba what he had to tell me.

He said, "Om Namah Shivaya[69]. Honor and worship your own Self. God dwells within you, as you."

The Five Aspects of Shiva

This is my take on a story I heard while hanging out at the ashram. I love this story and I hope that you enjoy it also.

Sometimes the Hindu god, Shiva, is pictured holding five objects. He has two legs and four arms to help him accomplish this feat. He stands on one leg. The objects he holds relate to the five aspects of the divine.

- God creates the world—without which there would be no play of consciousness.

- God maintains the world—without which there would be no continuous sense of self.

- God destroys the world—without which there would be no change and no growth.

- God hides himself within the world—without which there would be no drama.

- God reveals himself within the world—without which there would be no point.

The last aspect of God is also called grace. Since God is all-powerful, his hiding is perfect. We would never be able to see him if he did not allow it.

---

69 OM NAMAH SHIVAYA: (lit., Om, salutations to Shiva) The Sanskrit mantra of the Siddha Yoga lineage, known as the great redeeming mantra because some folk believe that it has the power to grant both worldly fulfillment and spiritual realization. OM (also written aum) is the primal sound from which the universe emanates; Namah is to honor or bow to; Shivaya denotes divine Consciousness, the Lord who dwells in every heart.

The first four aspects come from within us. The fifth aspect comes from outside us. An outer flame ignites our inner flame. Hence the need for the Guru!

Baba and Hello

As Baba became more famous, the Siddha Yoga Foundation established ashrams around the world. An ashram is a place people go to hang out with saints. Part of the ashram experience is greeting the Guru.

For a time I was privileged to sit near the front of the meditation room and watch people come up to meet the Guru. I watched hundreds of people approach and to each person, Baba said, "I welcome you with all my heart."

He was in no hurry. He seemed to take them in and hold them and cherish them. They may have exchanged a word or two or not. It was not important.

He had a scented peacock tail wand that he could wave in the face of a visitor. The unique smell could carry a person to rapture.

The message that seemed to be sent was, "I know who you really are. I welcome you totally and completely. You are safe here."

Near to Baba

One day at the ashram a visitor complained that Baba seemed to have the same group of seekers always around him. It was true that there always seemed to be a drive among the folk living in the ashram to get as close as possible to Baba's throne in the meditation hall so that we could be near him.

Baba responded, "These people try to sit near me because they think that they will get more of my attention. I am an old man and far-sighted. I am actually interested in and devoting my attention to those of you in the back of the hall."

The next day there was a push to seat ourselves as far back as possible.

Baba and Power

Unlike other paths toward our true nature like Hatha Yoga (The Position Path) or Karma Yoga (The Surrender path), Siddha Yoga (The Power path)[70] is supposed to achieve the results of inner peace through direct relationship with a being who dwells in such a place, a being who can perform miracles. Guru is formed from the Sanskrit words "Gu" which means darkness and "Ru" which means light. The Guru is the teacher that takes a student from darkness into light.

At an auditorium in front of several thousand people, Baba was asked by a questioner to perform a miracle. Baba responded, "I am constantly performing miracles. Even as I am speaking to you now, my beard is growing!"

Suddenly the mundane was sacred!

Baba and the Seekers

There seemed to be two kinds of people that showed up and found value at the ashram:

Some people showed up for whom life had turned into disaster; no matter what they were striving for it was beyond them. In helplessness they showed up and begged, "Please help me, I do not understand the world or my place in it. No matter what I attempt I fail to find happiness."

Other people showed up for whom life had turned into achievement; no matter what they were striving for it magically came to them. They seemed to easily collect fame, fortune, and good health. In helplessness they showed up and begged, "Please help me, I have mastered the world and my place in it, but no matter what I achieve I fail to find happiness."

---

70 These are my definitions. Here are more precise definitions: SIDDHA is spiritual energy (or power) experienced by a person in a state of enlightenment. A Siddha Guru is said to have the capacity to awaken the dormant spiritual energy of a disciple. HATHA YOGA consists of practices, both physical and mental, performed for the purpose of purifying and strengthening the body and mind. And KARMA is any action, be it physical, verbal, or mental, performed with the same goal in mind. In my opinion, selfless actions result when a person acts from a state of surrender to being of service to the world.

The message to both was the same. "Welcome home. You are loved and safe here."

Baba and My Baby

I was born several months premature and showed up on the planet at a birth weight, I am told, of only two and one-half pounds. I spent my first month here in a small heated box without human contact. At that time, many years ago, we did not know how important human contact is to an infant. To this day, I find comfort by pressing the back of my hand to a hard, flat surface.

I had wonderful parents who made me feel wanted and cherished as a child. But as an adult I kept going into relationships needing something. I could not seem to get enough physical contact. I have since learned that this position of neediness is common among preemies. I had a psychological hole and I was always looking for the sensations of human contact from someone else to fill it.

One day at the ashram, as I sat in meditation, it occurred to me that the adult me inside my head could go back into the story of my history and provide me the hugging and touching I had missed as an infant.

I found myself looking down at infant me in the hospital incubator. I reached in and picked me up. As I cradled me in my arms, I felt another presence.

I turned and discovered Baba standing beside me in his saffron robes. Without words he smiled and held out his hands for the baby. I handed infant me into his care.

He cradled infant me and as he did so I felt my adult self fill up with love from the inside much as a balloon fills up with air. I felt whole, healed, and complete.

Since that day, almost thirty years ago, I have never needed to seek another to feel loved. I have been happy to be at service to others and to provide whatever measure of love to them that I can give and that they are ready to receive. I have not needed anything back, not because my glass is half full, but because my glass is full to overflowing.

Thank you, Baba.

Baba's Gift

It came to pass that I, as a single parent, took my two young children in tow and traveled the United States in a car during the mid-seventies. At the start, our travel plan was to head from the San Francisco Bay Area up the coast to the World's Fair in Spokane and then to continue around the country during the remaining summer months.

I planned to leave sometime in the morning on a beautiful spring Saturday. At the time, I was in the practice of getting up fairly early (at least before the children stirred) and spending a half-hour in meditation.

During the meditation Baba appeared to me as a vision and said, "Stop by and see me on your way out of town." "Where shall I find you?" I asked. I am not really a joiner, and I was not actively following the comings and goings of the Guru. "Don't worry, I'll handle the arrangements." He said. And I found myself back, seated in my bedroom and starting the activities of my day.

As I finished loading the car and making a last goodbye tour of my apartment, I got a phone call from a spiritual friend. "I was just meditating and Baba appeared in front of me. He told me to contact you and give you his itinerary for today. He is staying at an ashram in Piedmont this weekend. It is a large home on a residential street. Here is the address."

The location was not far out of our way as we drove north. Hard to say no to so strong a message!

I showed up at the mansion with my two children, Ray, age seven and Mandy, age five. We walked into the main entry way and I said, "We are here to see Baba."

"Baba is not seeing anybody from the public today. He is holding only private conferences."

"I am here because I was asked to be here. A private conference will be fine with me. Let me know when he wishes to see me. My children and I will wait outside."

We sat together on a porch overlooking a garden of stone pathways, sculpted bushes, and ancient trees. We shared a snack of some trail mix. I loved being with my kids and luxuriating in the warm sunshine and cool breezes. This was so much better than the rushing, the traffic, and the road noise I had planned on experiencing at this time.

Eventually, I noticed that I had no particular agenda and no real attachment to actually getting in to see Baba. I was just following orders given me by some part of myself.

As I had this thought, a gentleman came out and found us on the porch. He informed me that I was late for my private appointment and that Baba was waiting.

We were escorted through a foyer containing a book sales table and into a large room. Baba was seated in a chair on a raised dais at the far end of the room. About thirty people were seated on cushions on the carpeted floor in front of him. I guess that when you are used to seeing thousands, thirty is private. I entered the room, where conversations were already in progress, and herded the children around the edge of the group to seat us in an open floor space to Baba's right.

We got settled with minimal disruption. I attempted to gather my wits about me. What the heck was I doing here? I was a stranger in a strange land and I had no clue as to how to behave or what to say. I began to observe the other folk for clues as to behavior.

A woman asked Baba to bless her and her family before they embarked on a trip. Bingo, when it was my turn I would ask Baba to bless my children and our upcoming adventure. No sooner had I thought this, than Baba turned and looked at me with a mischievous grin. He motioned to the children to come up to him. Ray had met Baba before (remember Davis) so he was unafraid. He led his sister up to the throne. Baba leaned forward and gave each of the children a handful of candy. In the Hindu belief system, candy from the Guru symbolizes blessings flowing from God into the world. I got my wish before I could express it.

I had to think fast. I remembered that when I was walking into the room a man was asking Baba to help him overcome an illness. It must be OK to ask for health and healing.

I had noticed that for the last few days as we were packing, Mandy had a little phlegm in her throat. I was worried that she might be coming down with a summer cold that would interfere with her enjoyment of our camping across the country. When it was my turn, I would ask the Guru to restore her to full health for the trip.

I had this thought just as Mandy was leaving Baba's dais with her piece of candy. Baba looked up at me over her head and again grinned his mischievous grin.

He reached out and around her with his right hand. He used the hand to scoop her back against him and cupped her back with his left hand. He then flicked the fingers of his right hand once against her chest, and set her back on her journey to me with a left hand push and pat on her shoulder. The interaction left her giggling as she reached me.

To my bemused amazement her breathing was clear and quiet as she sat there eating her candy. I could not know it at the time, but as it turned out, for the next two months of the summer we traveled without incident and camped all across the country. We did not have an insect bite, a rash, a sniffle or even a scratch that bled more than a minute. We needed no first aid although we traveled from campground to campground all across the states.

At one point, while inner tubing down the Spokane river, we took a break to sun ourselves, resting in only bathing suits in what turned out to be a patch of poison oak (I am a city boy). Some teenagers came along to tell us of our plight. We got back into the river and floated on. The river and the blessing removed all poison and we experienced no symptoms.

Six weeks later I dropped Mandy off at her mother's house in Cleveland and visited a couple I was friends with who lived in mid-Ohio. Bob, the man I was visiting, was a herbologist. As we walked through the Ohio woods he showed me a patch of Jewel Weed and explained that it was a Poison Ivy cure used by the Native Americans. It seems that in Ohio both Poison Ivy and Jewel Weed grow in similar locations so if you get exposed to one you have the cure handy in the other.

Over my protestations, he asked me to take a pocketful home with me. He said that something told him it would be useful for me to have. A few days later I showed up back in Cleveland to see Mandy. Her arm had broken out in several places with small running sores that looked like Poison Ivy. As I had been instructed, I made a poultice of the Jewel Weed and applied it to the spots on Mandy's arm. A few hours later the spots had dried up. There was no itching and no recurrence, as we continued together on our travels through Ohio and on to the New England states.

Meanwhile, here I am still sitting in the presence of the Guru and I have nothing to ask. I get back to watching the other visitors and hoping for inspiration. A college student goes up to Baba and asks him to autograph a copy of his recent book, *Guru*.

Baba has a stamp of his signature and takes great joy in inking the stamp and applying it to the flyleaf of the book. I decide that that would be sufficient interaction for me at this point. I see that the kids are happy eating their candy, so I get up and walk around to the back of the room and out to the book sales table. I buy a copy of "Guru" and attempt to sneak back to my place in the room.

As I enter the room with my new book, Baba looks up at me and motions me up to him. I approach and he leans forward and takes the book out of my numb hand.

He opens it and joyfully stamps his signature on it and shoves it back into my hands. He looks me in the eye and grins from ear to ear.

I am confronted with the Guru and I have nothing to say. I search desperately for some words and remember that I am in front of a Siddha Guru, said to be able to grant enlightenment with a single glance.

I look up at Baba and I start to form the sentence, "Baba, please grant me …" I get to the "me" in my mind and, as I search for my internal sense of self, I get lost.

I am me inside my head, then I am me in my body, then I am me throughout the room looking at Baba from thirty plus viewpoints at the same time, then I am a viewpoint that includes looking back at Alan and the room from Baba's position, then I expand through the walls of the room and the house. The engineer in me notes, with surprise that, rather than wall board, the outer wall of this old mansion consists of plaster then lathing then air space then exterior brickwork.

I experience the porch and the garden in which I had played earlier. Only this time my viewpoint includes looking through the eyes of squirrel on the branch of a tree, feeling the bark, smelling the air.

I expand to include the city block. I am in a kitchen making brunch; I notice the redness of my hands and consider putting cream on them later. I am a little girl, trying out my new roller skates and I hit a small bump in the sidewalk. I see, in a different grey-red spectrum, a cat movement that draws me to it with interest. I start as a dog notices me and, with a thrill, I leap away. Now I am driving down a shaded street; my hands tighten on the steering wheel as my foot moves off the gas, ready to hit my brakes as I see a little girl hesitantly skating on the sidewalk.

All this happens at the same time. All this is me. Somewhere I think, "How big am I?" and the expansion stops. I am the size of a city block and there is no center to me. Every part of me is equally me. Every part of me is interesting. I have lots of time to explore. I turn inward from my expanded border.

Part of me in an upstairs room of the ashram flashes a feeling of guilt as she notices that her meditation practice has slipped into a daydream. The links between each of my viewpoints seem to be made of bliss.

All my viewpoints have drama. All are full. I love and cherish each with a depth of feeling I had, up to now, only felt toward my children. Each viewpoint is the world to me. The Alan viewpoint, that I used to call home, is no more and no less important than any of the other viewpoints.

How long did this state last? In some sense only a breath, in some sense I am still there. Did you ever watch a movie and were so enthralled that it seemed to last only a moment but somehow two hours had passed? Later you could recall all the scenes, if not all the specific dialogue.

I would say the direct experience lasted what felt, after the fact, like ten minutes. It must have taken considerably less in clock time, perhaps only a breath or two.

With the "How long will this last?" thought, I was just in my Alan viewpoint, just looking in Baba's laughing eyes just looking in Alan's laughing eyes, patiently waiting for me to start and finish my sentence, "… grant me enlightenment."

Silly me! How can I form a coherent sentence about me when I have no clear idea of who I am?

I start to giggle …

ABOUT THE AUTHOR

Alan Weiner has been seeing hypnotherapy clients for the past 15 years. In addition to the training for his Clinical Hypnotherapist certification, Alan has studied and taught Neural-Linguistic Programming™ (NLP).[71]

Alan has made his living as a computer scientist, engineer, consultant, corporate manager, massage therapist, clinical hypnotherapist, public speaker, and technical writer. His hobbies include inventing, reading, visiting grandchildren, and training for triathlons. Alan lives in Newark, California with his wife Phoebe and his large dog, Max.

---

71 NLP is touched on in Chapter 9 when we discuss personal styles and in Chapter 11 when we discuss societal styles.

APPENDIX

COGNITIVE SCIENCE AND MEMORY FORMATION

This appendix provides a more technical background for some of the statements regarding mind-body interactions and memory formation that are made in a less formal manner throughout the book.

Cognitive science is the study of the nature of various mental tasks and the processes that enable them to be performed.[72] I consider it to be the scientific study of mind, intelligence, or consciousness. It draws from psychology, philosophy, neuroscience, linguistics, anthropology, computer science, biology, and physics.

Cognitive science, and in particular neuroscience, breaks memory into different types and sub-types located in different areas and structures of the brain.[73]

There are two main types of memory:

- Declarative "what" memory is the memory for facts and events that one can recall and declare. It has three sub-types:

  o Sensory—Sensory representation of events,

  o Episodic—Memory for past personally experienced events, and

  o Semantic—Memory for facts.

- Non-Declarative "how" memory is retrieved without conscious recollection. It has three sub-types:

  o Procedural memory—Action-oriented skills and operations,

  o Priming—Perceptual or conceptual skills, and

  o Conditioning—Repetition to develop non-declarative associations.

---

72 From The American Heritage Dictionary.

73 University of Memphis on-line course, *Neuropsychology/Behavioral Neuroscience*, by C J Long at http://neuro.psyc.memphis.edu/

I expand on some of these memory types below.

Procedural Memory

Procedural memory, also known as implicit memory, is the long-term memory of skills and procedures, or "how to" knowledge (procedural knowledge).

Procedural memory is often not easily verbalized. It can reflect simple stimulus-response actions or more extensive patterns learned over time. Examples of procedural memory are riding a bike, swimming, or reciting long poems. A procedural memory intervention was used to break up eating habit patterns in section 10.5.

Declarative memory

Declarative memory is the aspect of human memory that stores facts which can be discussed, or declared. It applies to standard textbook learning and knowledge, as well memories that we can remember in our mind's eye. There are two types of declarative memory:

- Semantic memory includes generalized knowledge that does not involve memory of a specific event. For instance, you can answer a question like "Is broccoli a fruit?" without remembering any specific time when you learned the difference between fruits and vegetables.

- Episodic memory refers to the memory of events, times, places, associated emotions, and other conception-based knowledge in relation to an experience. Hypnosis sessions often deal with early episodic memories.

Episodic Memory

Autobiographical memory is a type of episodic memory. Episodic memories can be likened to written stories.

Episodic memory is thought of as being a "one-shot" learning mechanism. You only need one exposure to an episode to remember it. Semantic memory, on the other hand, takes into consideration multiple exposures to similar events to extract a generalized rule. The semantic representation is updated on each exposure.

Episodic memory can be thought of as a "map" that ties together items in semantic memory. For example, semantic memory will tell you what your dog looks and sounds like. All episodic memories concerning your dog will reference this single semantic representation of "dog" and, likewise, all new experiences with your dog will modify your single semantic representation of your dog. This mechanism was discussed under "Chunking" in section 2.2.

Some researchers believe that you always remember episodic memories as episodic memories, while other researchers believe that episodic memories are refined into semantic memories over time. In this process, most of the episodic information about a particular event is generalized and the context of the specific events is lost. One modification of this view is that episodic memories which are recalled often are remembered as a kind of monologue. If you tell and re-tell a story repeatedly, you may feel that you no longer remember the event, but that what you're recalling has become your "story" of the event.

Emotion and episodic memory

The relationship between emotion and memory is complex, but generally, emotion tends to increase the likelihood that an event will be remembered later and that it will be remembered vividly. A memory may be laid down in great detail during a personally significant or shocking event. It can have a "photographic" quality. For example, a great many people can remember where they were when they heard of the terrorist attacks on September 11, 2001.

CLASSICAL I-STATEMENT CONSTRUCTION

The "I-Declaration" constructions used in this book are a special form of I-Statement developed by the author. They do not actually involve any other person and their primary goal is communication with self, not communication with other. I am not interested in changing anyone else's behavior.

On the other hand classical I-Statements can be used communicate with another person with the goal of changing their behavior. This is an approach taken in couple's therapy.

Properly constructed I-Statements avoid blaming, criticizing, judging, shaming, ridiculing and name-calling. They maintain a respectful attitude toward the receiver while assigning them the responsibility for change.

Historically an I-Statement has four parts:

1. "I"

2. what YOU feel or want

3. the event that evoked your feelings, and

4. the effect the event has on YOU.

These pieces combine to form a sentence as follows:

"I feel __#2__ when __#3__, because __#4__.

For example:

"I feel (2) hungry and crabby (3) when you are late home from work, because (4) I have waited to eat dinner with you."

To keep the communication an I-Statement:

-   Avoid Inserting "that" or "like"
    The phrases "I feel that …"-or "I feel like …" are really an opinion. "I feel" should always be followed by a feeling such as "sad," "glad," or "bad."

-   Avoid Disguised YOU-Statements
    These include sentences that begin with "I feel that you …" or "I feel like you …" You might as well just point your accusing finger at the person!

BIBLIOGRAPHY

Bandler, Richard; Grinder, John. *Frogs into Princes: Neuro-Linguistic Programming^{TM}*. Moab, Utah: Real People Press, 1979.

Bandler, Richard; Grinder, John. *Reframing: Neuro-Linguistic Programming^{TM} and the Transformation of Meaning*. Moab, Utah: Real People Press, 1982.

Bandler, Richard; Grinder, John. *Trance-Formations: Neuro-Linguistic Programming^{TM} and the Structure of Hypnosis*. Moab, Utah: Real People Press, 1981.

Beck, Don; Cowan, Chris. *Spiral Dynamics: Mastering Values, Leadership, and Change: Exploring the New Science of Memetics*. Cambridge, Massachusetts: Blackwell Business, 1996.

Boyne, Gil. *Transforming Therapy: A New Approach to Hypnotherapy*. Glendale, California: Westwood Publishing Company, 1989.

Cameron-Bandler, Leslie; Gordon, David; and Lebeau, Michael. *Know How: Guided Programs For Inventing Your Own Best Future*. San Rafael, California: FuturePace, Inc., 1985.

Clark, Sally. Maintains a website: www.sallyclarkmft.com.

Elman, Dave. *Hypnotherapy*. Glendale, California: Westwood Publishing Company, 1983.

Feldenkrais, Moshe. *Awareness Through Movement; Health Exercises for Personal Growth*. New York, New York: Harper & Row, 1972.

Gallo, Carmine. *10 Simple Secrets of the World's Greatest Business Communicators*. Naperville, Illinois: Sourcebooks, Inc., 2005.

Gilligan, Stephen. *Therapeutic Trances: The Cooperation Principle in Ericksonian Hypnotherapy*. New York, New York: Brunner/Mazel, Inc., 1987.

Grey, John. *Men are from Mars, Women are from Venus: A Practical Guide for Improving Your Communications and Getting What You Want in Your Relationships.* New York, New York: HarperCollins, 1992.

Gershon, David; Straub, Gail. *Empowerment: The Art of Creating Your Life as You Want It.* West Hurley, New York: High Point, 1989.

Harding, C. B. *Blue Collar Comedy Tour: The Movie.* Warner Brothers Pictures; 2003.

Harris, Thomas. *I'm OK, You're OK; a Practical Guide to Transactional Analysis.* New York, New York: Harper & Row, 1969.

Hayes, Steven; Smith, Specer. *Get Out of Your Mind & Into Your Life: The New Acceptance & Commitment Therapy.* Oakland, California: New Harbinger Publications, Inc., 2005.

Herbert, Frank. *Dune.* Philadelphia, Pennsylvania: Chilton Books, 1965.

Kubler-Ross, Elisabeth. *On Death and Dying.* New York, New York: Macmillan Publishing Company, 1969,

Levine, Stephen. *Who dies?: An Investigation of Conscious Living and Conscious Dying.* Garden City, New York: Anchor Press/Doubleday. 1982.

Louise-Diana. Gratitude First In All Things—Welcome from the Publisher. *Inner Fitness Living.* Vol. 28, November 2006.

Luskin, Frederic. *Forgive for Good: A Proven Prescription for Health and Happiness.* New York, New York: HarperCollins Publishers, Inc., 2002.

McGill, Ormand. *Hypnotism and Meditation: The Operational Manual for Hypnomeditation.* Glendale, California: Westwood Publishing Company, 1981.

Núñez, Rafael & Sweetser, Eve. (2006). With the Future Behind Them: Convergent Evidence From Aymara Language and Gesture in the Crosslinguistic Comparison of Spatial Construals of Time. *Cognitive Science*, 30(3), 401-450.

Paramhamsa, Muktananda. *GURU: Chitshaktivilas The Play of Consciousness.* New York, New York: Harper & Row, Publishers, Inc., 1971. This book has been republished in an expanded form as: *The Play of Consciousness (Chitshakti Vilas).* New York, New York: Harper & Row, Publishers, Inc., 1974.

Pert, Candace. *Molecules of Emotion: Why You Feel the Way You Feel.* New York, NY: Scribner, 1997.

Rivers, Dennis. *The Geometry of Dialogue: A Visual Way of Understanding Interpersonal Communication and Human Development.* This E-book is available for free download at www.newconversations.net, Third Edition, 2006

Stevens, Barry. *Burst Out Laughing.* Berkeley, California: Celestial Arts, 1984.

Tannin, Deborah. *You Just Don't Understand: Men and Women in Conversation.* New York, New York: Ballantine Books, 1991.

Tebbetts, Charles. *Self Hypnosis and Other Mind Expanding Techniques.* Dexter, Michigan: Thomson & Shore. Inc., 1989.

The American Heritage Dictionary of the English Language, Fourth Edition. Boston, Massachusetts: Houghton Mifflin Company, 2006.

The Holy Bible. New York, New York: Thomas Nelson & Sons, 1953.

Viorst, Judith. *Necessary Losses: The Loves, Illusions, Dependencies and Impossible Expectations that All of Us Have to Give Up in Order to Grow.* New York, New York: Ballantine Books, 1987.

Walsh, Brian. *Unleashing Your Brilliance: Tools & Techniques to Achieve Personal, Professional & Academic Success.* Victoria, BC: Walsh Seminars Ltd., 2005.

Glossary

Acceptance and Commitment Therapy (ACT): a therapy developed by Steven C. Hayes, a Professor of Psychology at the University of Nevada, Reno, that hinges on a distinction between pain and suffering.

Chunking: The mental process of association, integration, simplification, and assimilation that underlies learning. The word comes from a 1956 paper by George A. Miller, *The Magical Number Seven, Plus or Minus Two: Some Limits on our Capacity for Processing Information.*

Finger-drop technique: A technique for rapid self-hypnosis.

Goals that Grab: Goals formulated in such a way that they take on a life of their own. The goal setter is swept along by events as the world conspires to fulfill the goal.

I-Declaration: Fundamentally different than the classic I-Statement used in couple's therapy, the I-Declaration is used as a non-judgmental communication tool to define a level of clarity to one's self while avoiding the assignment of blame.

Joy visualization: An exercise designed to help 'reset' our interpretation of our situation in a more positive frame.

Mind: The collective aspects of intellect and consciousness. In this book the mind is modeled as having two parts. The conscious mind consists of everything that a person is aware of at any moment. The non-conscious mind consists of everything else. The conscious mind is limited to holding the 7+/-2 chunks of information while the non-conscious mind performs massive parallel processing and has no discernable limit.

Neural-Linguistic Programming™ (NLP): A set of models and principles used to describe the relationship between mind, language, and perception. Some NLP terms used in this book are:

Anchor: A signal associated with a feeling or state of being. Activating the anchor initiates the feeling.

Programs and meta-programs: The distinction between what we expect of ourselves and what we think the world expects of us.

Reframe: To look at a concept from a different point of view, to apply a different framework to the structure of a concept.

Thinking modalities: The way minds store sensory experience. The three main modalities are:

- visual (in the mind's eye)
- auditory (in the mind's ear)
- kinesthetic (in the body image)

Parts party: An internal dialogue that breaks our personality into many sub-personalities in order to identify parts that work together and parts that are in conflict. It is not that we are really fragmented; it is rather that we are trying to honor different rules for behavior that may be in conflict.

Trance state: An altered state of consciousness that lies at the border between the normal waking state and the normal sleep state. Aspects of the conscious and non-conscious mind may be brought together in this state. Two types of trance state are discussed in this book:

> **Meditation:** A self-induced trance state that has been practiced through the ages to bring peace, calm, and tranquility into the practitioner's life.

> **Self-hypnosis:** A self-induced trance that allows a practitioner to willfully communicate with his non-conscious mind to retrieve buried memories or suggest internal changes.

Useful Truths: Realizations that may or may not be true, but are manifestly useful.

978-0-595-69559-1
0-595-69559-0

CPSIA information can be obtained at www.ICGtesting.com
Printed in the USA
BVOW030122170413

318341BV00002B/41/A